The CAR of Nursing

By

Joe Robert Saye Komandan

Copyright © 2026

All rights reserved.

Published by:

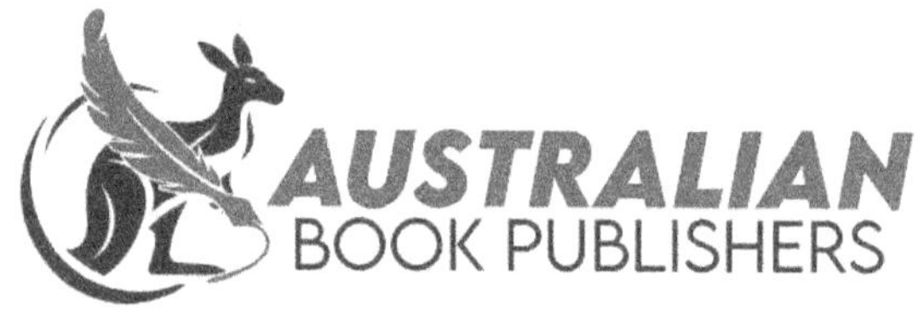

About the Author

Let me share a bit about my background. I was born in Nimba County, Liberia, West Africa, as one of nine children. Tragically, my father passed away when I was just six years old. I began school at the age of ten, but staying in class was often a struggle; my mother worked hard simply to put food on the table, let alone cover our school costs. In Year Four, I faced a major setback when I had to drop out because my mother couldn't afford the US$2.50 needed for my physical education T-shirt. I was frequently sent out of class while the other students remained, and the embarrassment of that experience stayed with me. It led me to realise that if I truly wanted an education, I would have to take ownership of my learning, something I began doing at age fourteen. From Year Four all the way through university, I had no financial support from my family for my education.

After finishing high school, I decided to pursue a career in teaching. I enrolled in a local teacher's college and eventually began teaching, dedicating seven years of my life to education in Africa before moving to Australia. Once in Australia, I explored different career paths and chose nursing, a field that was entirely new to me. My first step was completing a Certificate III in Aged Care, which I found deeply rewarding. While working at Blue Care as a personal care worker, I also began studying for a Diploma of Nursing. When I completed that diploma, I secured a position in a hospital and continued my studies by enrolling in a Bachelor of Nursing.

After graduating, I was thrilled to obtain a role as a clinical nurse, a position I've now held for about fifteen years. I'm currently working towards completing my master's degree in public health next year. Across my fifteen years in nursing, I've come to appreciate the incredible power of three simple yet valuable words, words that can be applied in any situation to save lives. This realisation inspired me to write my book, *The CAR of Nursing*.

Table of Contents

Introduction:
"The Car of Nursing"

Have you ever contemplated the unique experience of being in control of a vehicle that is more than an ordinary car, one that stands as a symbol of nursing excellence at its finest? Close your eyes and imagine a remarkable vehicle, meticulously crafted to carry you on an unparalleled journey through the enchanting world of healthcare. On this extraordinary voyage, you will witness the seamless fusion of empathy, expertise, and innovation, woven together to create a breathtaking masterpiece of restoration and wellbeing. I am about to guide you on a journey unlike any you've taken before, so please ensure your seatbelt is securely fastened as we prepare for this adventure.

Picture yourself standing before a polished, stunning vehicle, its brilliance catching the sunlight. Its exterior is adorned with symbols of healing and care, its body painted in vibrant colours that represent hope and dedication. As you approach, the door glides open, inviting you inside. The moment you settle into the plush seat, a sense of thrilling anticipation washes over you, making the experience truly unforgettable. You are being welcomed into the magical journey within the pages of *The Car of Nursing*. Let's set off together and discover what awaits us.

Before we dive into this exciting adventure, allow me to share a little about myself. My name is Joe Robert Saye-Komadan, and I am proud to be African Australian and a loving father of four. In my quest to uncover the hidden narratives of the nursing profession, I have spent countless years walking the corridors of hospitals, clinics, and medical institutions. As someone who deeply appreciates and documents the intricacies of human existence, I have been endlessly fascinated by the profound beauty that lies within the hearts and minds of those who devote themselves to the honourable calling of nursing.

The CAR of Nursing

Come with me on *The Car of Nursing* and experience the highs and lows of this extraordinary journey. Together, we will delve into the inner workings of the human body, revealing the intricate mechanisms that allow it to survive and thrive. We will explore the captivating history of nursing, from ancient civilisations to the modern day, where healers and caregivers have always played a vital role.

But this book goes deeper than facts and figures. My friend, it goes far beyond. *The Car of Nursing* honours the remarkable individuals who breathe life into the profession. By listening to nurses' stories of triumph and struggle, joy and sorrow, we gain a true understanding of the essence of nursing and its crucial role in holistic patient care.

Visualise yourself in a busy hospital ward, where the air is filled with beeping monitors and hushed conversations. Watch as a nurse gently holds the hand of a frightened patient, offering comfort in their darkest hour. Witness the unwavering dedication of a nurse working tirelessly through the night, feet aching, eyes determined, driven by the desire to make a difference.

Yet our exploration stretches far beyond hospital walls. We will uncover the many roles nurses play across society, from providing care in remote communities to offering vital support during disasters. Nurses are the unsung heroes who deliver healing to the world in ways we may never fully comprehend.

Prepare to be captivated by the stories in *The Car of Nursing*. They will inspire laughter, tears, and deep admiration for the resilience of the human spirit. Ready yourself for the courage and compassion of nurses across the globe. Get ready to be moved by the art and science of nursing, an incredible field that transforms lives.

So, dear reader, are you prepared to embark on this extraordinary adventure? Are you ready to explore the enchanting realm of nursing, to journey through discovery and enlightenment? If your answer is yes, then buckle up, this will be the ride of a lifetime. Welcome to the nursing journey, where love, healing, and humanity drive us forward.

The CAR of Nursing

Why is a career in nursing meaningful?

To truly understand nursing's importance, we must first explore its historical roots. Travel back in time with me as we uncover the origins and evolution of nursing care throughout the years.

In the early days of nursing, the concept of *care* was not clearly defined or emphasised. Nurses focused primarily on meeting patients' essential needs, administering medication, performing procedures, and providing physical comfort. While these aspects were vital, early nursing pioneers recognised the need for a more holistic approach, and so the true meaning of care began to emerge.

One of the greatest trailblazers in the development of modern nursing was Florence Nightingale. Widely regarded as the founder of the profession, Nightingale understood that nursing required more than treating physical illness. She recognised the importance of addressing a patient's psychological and emotional wellbeing, believing that care must encompass the whole person, not just their symptoms.

Nightingale's impact on nursing was profound. Her teachings laid the foundation upon which the modern nursing career was built. As I have come to understand it, the CAR of Nursing is a natural extension of Nightingale's core principles: maintaining a clean and healing environment, promoting health and preventative care, and recognising the significance of the nurse–patient relationship.

Fast forward to today, and we find ourselves in a healthcare system shaped heavily by technology, efficiency, and rapid clinical demands. While these innovations have greatly improved many aspects of care, they have also introduced challenges. Nurses often face increased responsibilities and significant time pressures, leaving limited space for the comprehensive, person-centred care that remains at the heart of our profession.

Despite these challenges, integrating the core of nursing, the CAR of Nursing, has never been more crucial. When holistic care is prioritised, patient outcomes improve markedly. By embracing these principles, nurses enrich the patient experience and contribute to stronger, more sustainable health outcomes.

One major benefit of incorporating the CAR of Nursing framework is its ability to address patients' emotional and psychological needs. Research consistently shows that patients who feel supported, heard, and understood experience better recovery rates and greater satisfaction with their care. Through emotional engagement, nurses can build trust and establish therapeutic relationships that go far beyond routine medical treatment.

Another vital strength of the CAR of Nursing lies in its emphasis on preventative care and health promotion. Nurses are uniquely positioned to educate, empower, and inspire patients to take charge of their health. By applying CAR principles, we can identify risk factors early, encourage healthy practices, and prevent chronic illnesses before they develop. This proactive approach not only saves lives but also significantly reduces long-term healthcare costs.

The CAR of Nursing also plays a crucial role in enhancing patient safety. When nurses prioritise the whole person, they are more attuned to subtle changes in a patient's condition and more likely to identify potential complications early. Through vigilant, attentive care, nurses can intervene promptly and prevent adverse events.

Beyond individual patient care, nursing profoundly influences the broader healthcare team. By fostering collaboration and open communication, nurses help create an environment where multidisciplinary professionals work seamlessly together. This team-based approach allows for more comprehensive assessment, coordinated treatment, and ultimately better outcomes for patients.

In conclusion, the care of nursing, and indeed the CAR of Nursing, is paramount in today's healthcare landscape. By embracing this framework, we strengthen the quality of care we provide, enhance the wellbeing of those we serve, and uphold the timeless principles established by Florence Nightingale. As a nurse, I am committed to integrating the CAR of Nursing into my practice and ensuring that every patient receives the highest standard of holistic care. Through this dedication, we continue to make a meaningful and lasting difference in the lives entrusted to us.

Introduction to the CAR of nursing:

Welcome to the world of nursing, where compassion and critical thinking come together to create meaningful and effective care. In this chapter, we will explore the concept of creative thinking and how it can be strengthened through the application of the CAR of Nursing. By using this professional framework, nurses can make sound, informed decisions, free from judgement based on opinions, assumptions, or vague statements.

The CAR framework equips nurses to navigate a wide range of situations, including problem-solving, innovation, and critical thinking in both professional and personal contexts. Together, we will embark on a journey to examine the six components of the CAR of Nursing: integrity, compassion, accountability, respect, engagement, and excellence.

Let's begin exploring how these principles shape not only our practice, but the very heart of nursing itself.

Integrity: The Foundation of Creative Thinking:

In nursing, integrity is the bedrock upon which our practice is built. When we approach problem-solving and innovation with integrity, we ensure that our actions remain aligned with our moral and ethical principles. Nurses who uphold integrity place patient safety and wellbeing above all else. By incorporating this component into the CAR of Nursing, we establish a strong, trustworthy foundation upon which creative thinking can flourish.

Compassion: Empathy Fuels Innovation:

Compassion is a driving force in nursing, fuelling our ability to empathise with others. As we engage in problem-solving and critical thinking, we must consider the perspectives of those affected by our decisions. By consciously applying compassion within the CAR of

Nursing, we unlock our creative potential and develop solutions that genuinely address the needs and concerns of all involved.

Accountability: Vital aspects in nursing:

Accountability is a vital aspect of the CAR of Nursing and extends beyond our professional lives into our personal and family relationships. It involves taking responsibility for our actions, behaviours, and decisions. By holding ourselves accountable, we demonstrate our commitment to being reliable and trustworthy individuals. This, in turn, fosters a sense of security and stability within our relationships, as our loved ones can depend on us to honour our commitments and fulfil our roles within the family.

Respect: Valuing Diverse Perspectives:

The threads of respect weave through every interaction in nursing, creating a strong and cohesive fabric of care. Diverse perspectives are essential when engaging in creative thinking. By incorporating this component into the CAR of Nursing, we recognise the importance of valuing and respecting the thoughts and opinions of others. When we actively listen and honour differing viewpoints, we open ourselves to new ideas and innovative solutions that may otherwise have eluded us.

Engagement: Active Participation in Problem-Solving:

Engagement represents active participation within the CAR of Nursing. When we fully engage with the challenges before us, we immerse ourselves in meaningful problem-solving and critical thinking. This level of involvement enables us to uncover hidden insights and explore alternative approaches. By engaging with our creativity, we tap into our full potential, leading to more effective and innovative solutions.

Excellence: Striving for the Best:

In nursing, excellence is an aspiration that drives us to provide the highest standard of care possible. By incorporating excellence into the CAR of Nursing, we set our sights on finding optimal solutions that lead to positive outcomes. Striving for excellence means going above and beyond, continually seeking improvement and embracing opportunities for growth. Through this commitment, we unlock the full potential of our creative abilities.

Applying the CAR Framework:

Now that we've explored the six components of the CAR of Nursing, let's turn our attention to applying this framework to problem-solving, innovation and critical thinking across different areas of life. The strength of this approach lies in its ability to guide us through a clear, step-by-step process, ensuring that we tackle challenges systematically, deliberately and effectively.

The (C) Concern: Contextualising the Problem:

The first step in the CAR framework is identifying and understanding the concern. Concerns or contexts can appear in many forms and should never be overlooked. Recognising and acknowledging them allows us to explore the root causes of a problem and develop practical, appropriate solutions. By engaging our emotional intelligence, we gain valuable insight into the issues that need our attention. Concerns may be physical, emotional, spiritual or intuitional, and it would be naive to ignore any of them, whether in healthcare or in everyday life.

The (A) stands for Action: Taking Necessary Steps:

Once the concerns have been identified, it is time to act. This step involves both assessment and intervention. By thoroughly assessing the situation, we gather relevant information and gain a clear understanding of the problem. With this knowledge, we can take the necessary steps to address the concern directly. Acting is a dynamic process that calls for critical thinking and creativity, as nurses must consider multiple factors and potential outcomes in their decision-making.

The (R) stands for Result: Evaluating the Outcome.

The final step in the CAR framework is to evaluate the result. By carefully assessing the outcome of our actions, we can determine how effective our problem-solving and critical-thinking strategies have been. Results may vary, and it is important to remain open-minded and adaptable. If the desired outcome isn't achieved, we can use this as an opportunity to reflect, learn and refine our approach. The feedback we gain from our results becomes a valuable guide for future problem-solving endeavours.

Application of the Car of Nursing:

The CAR of Nursing can be effectively applied not only in healthcare settings but also in our personal lives. Nursing principles and skills are highly transferable, enabling us to solve problems and make informed decisions well beyond the traditional boundaries of healthcare.

For example, imagine facing a challenge that calls for critical thinking and problem-solving. By applying the CAR of Nursing, we begin by contextualising the concern and gaining a full understanding of its implications. We then identify and implement the steps needed to address the challenge. Finally, we evaluate the outcome, reflecting on the effectiveness of our approach and making adjustments where necessary. Through this process, we unlock our creative potential and use critical thinking to overcome personal obstacles.

Conclusion:

In conclusion, the CAR of Nursing is a powerful tool for unlocking creative potential, enhancing critical thinking and fostering innovation in problem-solving. Through the six components, integrity, compassion, accountability, respect, engagement and excellence, nurses can navigate complex challenges in a systematic and effective way. By applying the CAR framework of Concern, Action and Result, we are able to tackle problems head-on, using creativity and critical thinking to guide our decisions.

Whether in healthcare settings or in our personal lives, the CAR of Nursing empowers us to make informed choices and develop innovative solutions that support holistic care. By embracing the CAR of Nursing as both a professional and personal tool, we unlock our full potential and drive positive change in every aspect of our lives.

Chapter 1:
Applying the Car of Nursing in Practice

The first letter of the Car of Nursing is **C**, which stands for **Concern** or **Context**. This initial step helps us identify the issue or problem at hand. I vividly recall a time when a patient came in with a high fever and complained of severe abdominal pain while I was working in the emergency department. My primary concern was to assess the severity of the pain and address the underlying cause. By understanding the context of the patient's symptoms, I could focus my actions and deliver appropriate care.

The second letter is **A**, which stands for **Action** or **Assessment**. This step involves taking suitable actions or evaluating the situation to provide the best care. In the case of the patient with abdominal pain, I immediately conducted a thorough physical assessment. I observed their vital signs, listened to their abdomen for abnormal sounds, and asked detailed questions about their symptoms. These actions enabled me to gather the necessary information to make an informed treatment decision.

Once the necessary actions have been taken and the appropriate care implemented, it is essential to evaluate the outcomes. This brings us to the final letter of the CAR of Nursing, **R**, which stands for **Result** or **Report**. Assessing the consequences of our actions is a critical step in patient care. It allows us to learn from our experiences and make adjustments to enhance the patient's well-being. In the case of the patient with abdominal pain, I closely monitored their vital signs and conducted regular assessments to evaluate the effectiveness of the treatment. I tracked the outcomes, ensured the patient responded positively to the interventions, contacted the treating doctor promptly, and completed the relevant documentation.

The CAR of Nursing highlights the importance of its components: **Integrity, Compassion, Accountability, Respect, Engagement,** and **Excellence** in delivering holistic care. As nurses, we must demonstrate trust, authenticity, truthfulness, and transparency, while striving for equality.

Integrity forms the foundation of our profession and is essential for building trust with our patients. **Compassion** drives us to provide care with kindness, empathy, and support. Through compassion, we can create a healing environment for our patients.

Accountability is another crucial aspect of nursing. Nurses are responsible for our actions, behaviours, and decisions. We must take ownership of the care we provide and continuously strive for excellence. This involves being open to feedback, reflecting on our practice, and making improvements as necessary. By holding ourselves accountable, we ensure we consistently deliver high-quality care.

Respect is fundamental in nursing. We must create a safe and inclusive environment for our patients, honouring their privacy, opinions, and cultural beliefs. We should also extend this respect to our colleagues and interdisciplinary team members, fostering a collaborative and supportive working environment. Similarly, engagement is essential in nursing. We must be team players, resourceful, and willing to lend a helping hand to our colleagues. By actively engaging in our practice, we contribute to our peers' growth and development and promote camaraderie within the healthcare team.

Finally, **Excellence** is a cornerstone of nursing. We should empower others, inspire, and adopt innovative approaches to patient care. Excellence is not merely about meeting standards; it is about going above and beyond to deliver exceptional care. By embodying excellence, we can make a lasting impact on the lives of our patients and their families.

The CAR of Nursing emphasises the importance of completing all the letters (C, A, R) to form a complete framework. Omitting any of these steps can lead to errors, self-blame, and negative outcomes. By embracing the CAR of Nursing, we can ensure thorough and well-rounded patient care.

The CAR of Nursing

The CAR of Nursing is not only applicable in healthcare environments but also serves as a valuable tool in our personal lives for problem-solving and thoughtful decision-making. Its principles extend beyond hospital walls and can be used in various situations, such as responding to patient needs, addressing concerns, and highlighting potential risks.

Emotional intelligence is vital in recognising issues and taking appropriate actions. As nurses, we need to tap into our emotional awareness, paying attention to our feelings and those of others. This connection enables us to form a deep relationship with our patients and approach their concerns with empathy and compassion.

Applying the CAR (Concern, Action, Result) framework in nursing reduces the likelihood of regrets and enhances patient safety and well-being. This framework serves as a guide, ensuring healthcare providers consistently deliver comprehensive care tailored to patients' needs. By adhering to CAR principles, professionals can be confident they have taken every necessary step to facilitate positive outcomes.

In conclusion, the CAR of Nursing represents a vital instrument that fosters providing holistic care to patients. By embracing the principles of Concern, Action, and Result, healthcare professionals can make informed decisions that address the diverse needs of patients. Furthermore, the CAR of Nursing underscores the significance of integrity, compassion, accountability, respect, engagement, and excellence within clinical practice. It directs practitioners in their commitment to quality care while safeguarding patient welfare. Consequently, let us collectively embrace the potential of the CAR of Nursing in our professional practice, striving to effectuate a meaningful impact in the lives of those we serve.

The CAR of Nursing in Professional Development

To fully grasp the significance of the Car of Nursing, it is essential to delve into its acronym, CAR, which stands for **Concern, Action,** and **Result**. This framework is both simple and powerful, serving as a guiding principle that enables proactive problem-solving rather than reactive responses.

The CAR of Nursing

Nurses encounter a wide range of challenges daily. These challenges may include providing high-quality patient care amid complex medical conditions, managing interpersonal conflicts among team members, or navigating intricate ethical dilemmas related to patient rights and healthcare policies. Each situation demands a thoughtful and structured approach to ensure positive outcomes.

The CAR of Nursing equips us with a comprehensive toolkit and a proactive mindset needed to effectively address these challenges. By identifying specific concerns, devising informed actions, and evaluating outcomes, nurses can ensure optimal care while fostering a collaborative and ethical work environment. This framework enhances clinical practice and promotes personal and professional growth within the nursing profession.

Integrity forms the foundation of the CAR of Nursing, reflecting the essential values nurses must uphold. Trust, authenticity, truthfulness, and transparency should be deeply embedded in our professional identity. These values are crucial for building strong relationships with patients and colleagues, creating an environment characterised by respect and open communication. By adhering to high standards of integrity, we facilitate ethical decision-making and deliver compassionate care. Building integrity means being honest, even when no one is watching. Think about your relationships: How often do you value them without your partner? Have you gone the extra mile for someone you love? Reflect on your daily actions, do they genuinely align with the values you stand for?

Compassion, recognised as the second component of the CAR of Nursing, is our profession's foundation. It embodies the essence of providing care through kindness, empathy, and unwavering support. This approach is a professional obligation, so it is crucial to follow this procedure.

The interactions we have with patients are extraordinarily significant and have the potential to create a profound effect on their emotional and physical well-being, making each interaction a critical part of their care. By consistently practising compassion, we cultivate a supportive and restorative environment where patients can find solace and healing during challenging times.

In today's rapidly evolving healthcare environment, where increasing demands may compromise genuine patient interaction, healthcare providers must dedicate time to connect with patients on a meaningful personal level. This involves delivering clinical care while actively listening to their concerns, understanding their fears, and offering reassurance. Such meaningful interactions create bonds of trust and respect that facilitate healing. Reflecting on your everyday life, consider how much time you allocate to listening, caring for, and demonstrating kindness to those you cherish. Just as we strive to connect with our patients, it is equally important to nurture our relationships with loved ones, ensuring that compassion remains a core value in all aspects of life.

Accountability, the third component of the CAR of Nursing, ensures we take ownership of our actions, behaviours, and decisions. As healthcare professionals, we hold tremendous responsibility, and being accountable means acknowledging and learning from our mistakes. Through self-reflection and continuous improvement, we can provide the best possible care to our patients.

Respect, the fourth component of the Car of Nursing, emphasizes the importance of valuing our patients' individuality and autonomy. Respecting their privacy, opinions, and cultural backgrounds is not just an ethical obligation and an essential aspect of patient-centred care. By creating a safe and inclusive environment, patients are empowered to actively participate in their care and make informed decisions.

Engagement, the fifth component, involves teamwork and resourcefulness in practice. Collaboration with colleagues, interdisciplinary teams, and patients is paramount in delivering comprehensive care. By actively engaging in our profession, seeking opportunities for professional growth, and embracing lifelong learning, we cultivate an environment of excellence.

Excellence, the sixth and final component of the CAR of Nursing, encourages us to continually strive for the highest standards of care. Pursuing excellence means providing evidence-based practices, empowering others, inspiring them, and fostering a culture of innovation. Through our commitment to excellence, we elevate the nursing profession and genuinely make a difference in the lives of our patients.

The CAR of Nursing is not confined to healthcare settings; its principles extend into our personal lives. Its principles can be instrumental in solving everyday problems, making sound decisions, and fostering individual growth. When faced with challenges outside of work, the Car of Nursing offers a framework for approaching them with integrity, compassion, and excellence.

Emotional intelligence plays a critical role in applying the CAR of Nursing effectively. Being self-aware, empathetic, and able to perceive and manage our own emotions and those of others allows us to identify concerns and take appropriate actions. Emotional intelligence is the driving force that propels the CAR of Nursing forward, allowing us to provide holistic care.

In summary, the CAR of Nursing is not just a catchy acronym; it represents a philosophy that guides us in delivering holistic care and making sound decisions. Its components, integrity, compassion, accountability, respect, engagement, and excellence, propel us forward and define our professional identity. By embracing the principles of CAR, we create a solid foundation for personal and professional growth, effective decision-making, and career progression in nursing.

Reflecting on my journey within the CAR of Nursing, I am reminded of the countless patients I have encountered throughout my career. Each individual, with their own unique concerns and needs, reinforces the importance of CAR in every aspect of our practice. The Car of

The CAR of Nursing

Nursing is not just a vehicle to be driven but a vessel that carries us towards positive change, empowerment, and meaningful connections.

The following chapters will explore how the CAR of Nursing can be integrated into daily practice. We will hear stories from fellow nurses who have embraced these principles and witnessed their profound impact on professional development. Together, let us embark on a journey towards excellence, compassion, and growth as we uncover the true potential of the CAR of Nursing.

The CAR of Nursing in Family and Personal Life

As I delved deeper into exploring how the principles of the Car of Nursing can be applied to improve relationships, communication, and decision-making in personal and family life, I realised the tremendous impact these principles can have on our daily interactions. The acronym **CAR (Concern, Action, Result)** is a powerful tool to guide us towards making sound decisions that benefit both ourselves and those around us. Here are some real-life examples of positive outcomes:

Strengthening Relationships: Imagine a couple facing a disagreement or a shared challenge. Rather than resorting to heated arguments or dismissive comments, they approach the situation with concern and genuine curiosity. One partner might ask thoughtful questions, such as, "Can you help me understand why you feel this way?" This opens the door to meaningful dialogue and encourages others to express their feelings more fully.

As the conversation progresses, they acknowledge each other's perspectives, affirming feelings with statements like, "I can see why this matters so much to you." This validation fosters empathy and creates a sense of safety and respect. After exploring each other's views, they collaborate to identify a compromise that respects both sides. They might say, "Let's brainstorm some solutions that can work for both of us." This cooperative approach resolves the immediate concern and strengthens their bond, leading to greater trust and emotional closeness. Through this process, they enhance their communication skills and deepen their understanding of one another, ultimately fostering a healthier and more resilient relationship.

Improving Workplace Dynamics: In a team meeting, instead of dismissing a colleague's idea, a leader applies concern or curiosity by asking, "Can you explain your thought process behind this idea?" The leader's actions or acknowledges their effort and input, saying, "I appreciate the creativity you've put into this." Then, with a constructive result or Response, they discuss how the idea can be refined or aligned with the project. Such interactions can boost morale and innovation.

Resolving Conflicts in Parenting: A parent applying CAR might approach a child's frustration with concern or curiosity, asking, "What's making you upset right now?" They act by acknowledging the child's feelings: "It's okay to feel frustrated, it happens to all of us." Their result involves brainstorming solutions together, fostering safety and open communication in the parent-child relationship.

Effective Decision-Making: Suppose a community group is planning a new project. Members apply the CAR approach to understand diverse viewpoints. By Acknowledging each perspective and responding constructively, they achieve consensus more smoothly, ensuring everyone feels valued. The CAR approach emphasises active listening, empathy, and collaboration, transformative tools in various settings.

Integrity is the first principle that comes to mind when discussing the CAR of Nursing. It is the foundation upon which trust and honesty thrive. In personal and family life, it is essential to uphold integrity and to always stay true to our values and principles. Doing so creates a safe and reliable environment where open communication and meaningful connections can flourish.

Compassion is highly valued in nursing and can greatly enhance relationships and communication in personal life. It involves showing empathy, understanding, and genuine care. When we approach others with compassion, we create space for them to feel heard and respected, fostering connection and understanding within our relationships.

Accountability is a vital aspect of the Car of Nursing that applies to personal and family life. It is about taking responsibility for our actions, behaviours, and decisions. We demonstrate our commitment to being reliable and trustworthy individuals by holding ourselves accountable. This fosters a sense of security and stability within our relationships, as our loved ones can rely on us to fulfil commitments and roles within the family.

Respect is a fundamental principle in personal life. Showing respect for others' privacy and opinions creates an atmosphere of trust and acceptance. It is crucial to recognize and appreciate the uniqueness of everyone in our family and respect their boundaries. By doing so, we foster an environment where open and honest communication can thrive, allowing for the free exchange of thoughts and ideas without judgment or criticism.

Engagement is an essential principle that encourages active participation and involvement in personal and family life. It requires us to be present and fully committed to our relationships. By engaging wholeheartedly with our loved ones, we show them that they are a priority in our lives. This can involve actively participating in family discussions, attending important events, or simply spending quality time together without distractions. Through engagement, we strengthen the bonds that hold us together as a family.

Excellence, the final principle, inspires us to aim for the highest standards in personal and family life. It involves continuously seeking opportunities for growth and improvement. By aiming for excellence within our relationships and communication, we set the stage for personal and collective growth. This can be achieved by actively seeking knowledge and resources that enable us to be the best versions of ourselves. It also involves setting goals and challenges for us and our family, pushing the boundaries of what we believe we can achieve.

The CAR of Nursing

Throughout this exploration, I also recognised the importance of **empowering others** and inspiring innovation. Empowering our loved ones to take charge of their own lives and make decisions that align with their goals and aspirations not only promotes personal growth but also strengthens our relationships. By fostering a culture of innovation within our families, we encourage creativity and problem-solving, helping us navigate through the challenges that life may throw at us.

In conclusion, the CAR of Nursing provides a comprehensive framework to enhance relationships, communication, and decision-making in personal and family life. By embodying integrity, compassion, accountability, respect, engagement, excellence, empowerment, and innovation, we can create loving and supportive environments where each member feels valued and heard. It is through the application of these principles that we can forge deeper connections, improve communication, and make sound decisions that ultimately contribute to our overall well-being and happiness. Let us embrace the CAR of Nursing and embark on a journey toward stronger, more fulfilling personal and family lives.

Chapter 2:
The Components of the Car of Nursing

Integrity: The Foundation of Nursing

To build trust with our patients, we must be honest and transparent in our interactions. This means communicating openly, sharing important information, and being upfront about potential risks and challenges. Patients rely on us to provide accurate information so they can make informed decisions about their healthcare. By displaying integrity in our communication, we establish a foundation of trust that forms the basis of a strong nurse–patient relationship.

Being authentic is equally important in nursing. When we are authentic, we are genuine and true to ourselves, both as individuals and as healthcare professionals. Patients can sense when someone is being disingenuous, and it can erode the trust they place in us. By embracing our own values and beliefs and staying true to them, we demonstrate authenticity and earn the respect of our patients and colleagues.

Integrity also means striving for equality in our practice. It requires treating all patients with respect and dignity, regardless of their background, social status, or beliefs. In nursing, we are advocates for our patients' rights, ensuring they receive fair and unbiased treatment. By practising integrity in this way, we contribute to a more just and compassionate healthcare system.

But integrity in nursing isn't limited to our professional lives. It extends beyond the hospital walls and into our personal lives as well. It means living with integrity in all aspects of life, being accountable for our actions, and upholding the values we hold dear. Our patients trust us to be their advocates and caregivers, and we must always strive to be worthy of that trust.

Compassion: The Heart of Nursing: Caring for Self and Others

Compassion is at the heart of nursing. It is the ability to truly care for others, to empathise with their pain and suffering, and to offer them comfort and support. But compassion doesn't stop at caring for our patients; it includes caring for ourselves as well. To effectively care for others, we must also prioritise self-care and ensure that our own needs are met.

Self-care is not selfish; it is necessary for our well-being. Nursing is a demanding profession, both physically and emotionally, and it can take a toll on us if we neglect our own needs. By prioritising self-care, we are better able to show up for our patients with compassion and empathy. Taking the time to rest, recharge, and engage in activities that bring us joy and fulfilment allows us to be the best version of ourselves for our patients.

Kindness, empathy, and supportiveness are qualities all nurses should possess. These qualities enable us to connect with our patients on a deeper level, to listen to their concerns, and to provide the emotional support they need. In moments of crisis or vulnerability, our compassion can make a world of difference, offering solace and hope during challenging times.

To truly understand the role of compassion in nursing, we must delve into its historical roots. Compassion has always been an integral part of the profession, dating back to the days of Florence Nightingale. She was not only a pioneer in the field of nursing but also a champion of compassionate care. For Nightingale, compassion meant recognising the individuality and inherent worth of each patient, and providing care that went beyond the physical.

In the early days of nursing, compassion was often expressed through simple acts of kindness, such as holding a patient's hand, listening to their concerns, or offering words of comfort. These small gestures had a profound impact, helping patients feel seen, heard, and cared for. Over time, however, compassion in nursing evolved to encompass not just acts of kindness but also a deeper understanding of the emotional and psychological needs of patients.

Research has shown that compassion is not just a pleasant gesture; it is a vital component of effective patient care. Studies demonstrate that when patients perceive their nurses as compassionate, they report higher levels of satisfaction and experience improved health outcomes. This highlights the importance of compassionate care in promoting healing and facilitating recovery.

But how do nurses prioritise and cultivate compassion within themselves? The answer lies in self-care. As healthcare providers, we are often so focused on caring for others that we neglect our own well-being. Yet, to provide truly compassionate care, we must first care for ourselves. Through self-care, we replenish our inner reservoirs of compassion, allowing us to extend it meaningfully to others.

Self-care encompasses physical, emotional, and spiritual well-being. Engaging in activities that promote physical health, such as regular exercise, a balanced diet, and sufficient sleep, is crucial. Taking time away from work, engaging in hobbies, and connecting with loved ones supports emotional resilience. Nurturing spiritual well-being through meditation, prayer, or activities that bring joy and meaning also contributes to the cultivation of compassion.

Nurses must also possess certain qualities to effectively demonstrate compassion. Kindness, empathy, and support are essential traits that help us connect with patients on a deeper level. Being present and attentive, listening with an open heart, and validating patients' emotions and experiences are key components of compassionate care.

Moreover, compassion in nursing extends beyond interactions with patients. It includes the way we communicate and collaborate with colleagues, and the ways we support and uplift one another. By fostering a culture of compassion within the profession, we create a safe and supportive environment for both patients and healthcare providers.

In day-to-day practice, compassion can be expressed through small but meaningful acts. Taking the time to sit with a patient and hold their hand, offering a genuine smile, or taking a few extra moments to explain a procedure can make a world of difference to someone who may be feeling vulnerable or anxious. These acts demonstrate our commitment to seeing patients as unique individuals, not merely as medical cases.

The practice of compassion in nursing also involves recognising and acknowledging our own limitations. It is important for nurses to accept that they cannot always fix every problem or alleviate every pain. However, even in the face of challenges, we can still provide compassionate care by showing empathy, offering support, and advocating for our patients.

Compassion is not reserved solely for times of illness or vulnerability. It extends to all aspects of nursing, including health promotion and disease prevention. By empowering patients with knowledge, helping them navigate healthcare systems, and encouraging them to take an active role in their own well-being, we demonstrate our commitment to compassionate care.

In conclusion, compassion is the beating heart of nursing. It is a fundamental quality that enhances patient care, fosters empathy, and creates a safe and supportive environment. As nurses, we must prioritise self-care, cultivate essential qualities such as kindness and empathy, and embrace compassion as an integral part of our practice. By doing so, we not only enhance the well-being of our patients but also enrich our own lives and the interconnected nature of the nursing community. Let us never forget that compassion is not just a feeling, but an action that has the power to heal and transform lives.

Accountability: Taking Responsibility in Nursing

Throughout the history of nursing, accountability has always been a cornerstone of the profession. From the early days of Florence Nightingale to the modern healthcare system we have today, nurses have been held accountable for their actions and their impact on patient care. Accountability has evolved over time as our understanding of patient safety and professional conduct has grown.

In the early days of nursing, accountability was mainly focused on ensuring that the basic needs of patients were met. Nurses were responsible for providing comfort, cleanliness, and nutrition. They had to be diligent in their duties, ensuring patients received the care they needed in a timely manner. This sense of accountability was driven by a desire to improve patient outcomes and ensure the well-being of those in our care.

As healthcare professionals, we have a moral and ethical responsibility to be accountable for our actions, behaviours, and decisions. Accountability in nursing is not just about following rules and protocols; it is about taking ownership of our role in providing safe and effective care to our patients. But accountability extends beyond our individual actions; it also involves holding others accountable and advocating for a culture of safety within our healthcare organisations. This means speaking up when we witness unsafe practices or unethical behaviour and ensuring that our concerns are addressed. By being accountable, we contribute to a safe and supportive environment for both patients and healthcare professionals.

Patient safety is paramount in nursing, and being accountable ensures that we are doing everything in our power to protect our patients from harm. It means taking responsibility for our actions and seeking to learn from any mistakes or missteps that may occur. As nurses, we must continually reflect on our practice, seek feedback, and engage in lifelong learning to improve our skills and knowledge.

As healthcare advanced and nursing became more specialised, the concept of accountability expanded. Nurses were not only responsible for the physical care of their patients, but also for their emotional and psychological well-being. Patient safety became a central focus, and nurses were held accountable for providing a safe environment. This included everything from ensuring proper medication administration to preventing hospital-acquired infections.

In recent years, accountability in nursing has taken on a new meaning, as our understanding of patient safety and professional conduct has deepened. It is no longer enough to complete tasks and provide physical care. Nurses must also be accountable for their interactions with patients and colleagues. This includes being mindful of cultural differences and treating all patients with respect and dignity. It means striving for equality in healthcare and advocating for the rights of our patients.

The CAR of Nursing

Accountability also extends to our own personal and professional development. As nurses, we must be accountable for our learning and growth. We must stay current with evidence-based practices and continually seek opportunities to improve our skills and knowledge. This ensures that we provide the best possible care to our patients and remain at the forefront of our profession.

In my practice, I have embraced the concept of accountability wholeheartedly. I understand that my actions directly impact patient safety and the overall quality of care provided. I strive to be a trustworthy and authentic nurse, always acting in the best interests of my patients. Transparency is also crucial to accountability. I am open and honest with my patients, explaining the reasoning behind my actions and involving them in their care decisions.

One aspect of accountability that I find particularly important is the responsibility to respond to patient needs promptly. This means being efficient and organised in my work, but also attentive and compassionate. Patients deserve to have their concerns addressed promptly and receive the care they need when they need it. By being accountable in this way, I can build a strong rapport with my patients and provide them with the best possible experience.

Accountability also extends to my interactions with colleagues. As a nurse, I recognise that I am part of a team and that we all share responsibility for patient care. I am accountable for offering support to my colleagues, sharing information and best practices, and collaborating to ensure the best outcomes for our patients. By fostering a culture of accountability within our team, we can provide seamless and coordinated care.

Overall, the concept of accountability is essential to ensuring the delivery of holistic care in nursing. It is not just about being responsible for our actions, but about recognising the impact we have on patient safety and the overall quality of care. By embracing accountability, we can provide the best possible care to our patients and contribute to the advancement of the nursing profession. In my own practice, I will continue to prioritise accountability and strive to improve the care I provide each day.

Respect: Creating a Culture of Dignity in Nursing

In healthcare, respect is the foundation of the entire system. As a nurse, I understand the profound significance of respect in nurturing a safe and inclusive environment for patients and healthcare professionals. It is an intangible power that holds the potential to transform lives and shape the future of healthcare.

Respect is a fundamental value in nursing. It is the cornerstone of professionalism, ensuring we provide a safe and supportive environment for our patients. Respect encompasses a range of behaviours, from valuing individuals' privacy and opinions to demonstrating professionalism both at work and beyond it.

In nursing, we are entrusted with caring for individuals at their most vulnerable moments. Respecting their privacy means protecting their personal information and maintaining confidentiality. It means seeking their consent and involving them in their care decisions. By respecting their autonomy and dignity, we empower our patients and honour their individuality.

Respect also means treating our colleagues with professionalism and courtesy. Collaboration and teamwork are essential in healthcare, and by respecting the expertise and contributions of our colleagues, we can achieve better outcomes for our patients. It means valuing diversity and recognising the unique strengths that each member of the healthcare team brings to the table.

One cannot discuss respect without acknowledging the importance of patients' privacy and opinions. In the evolution of nursing practice, privacy has emerged as a fundamental right for every individual seeking healthcare. Professional privacy ensures that we honour the sanctity of our patients' personal information and uphold a high standard of confidentiality. By creating an environment where patients feel secure and protected, we establish a strong foundation of trust between caregivers and patients.

Furthermore, respecting patients' opinions is vital in nursing practice. Each patient brings a unique perspective and a personal understanding of their health. Our duty as healthcare providers is to listen attentively to their voices and honour their autonomy. By actively engaging in shared decision-making, we empower patients to take charge of their health, fostering a sense of ownership and accountability.

Promoting respect in the nurse–patient relationship is an ongoing endeavour that involves active listening and open communication. Active listening, where we fully immerse ourselves in the patient's words, reveals insight into their concerns, hopes, and fears. By truly hearing them, we offer validation and acknowledge their worth as individuals. Open communication is equally essential, helping create an atmosphere of trust where patients feel comfortable expressing their thoughts and concerns without fear of judgement.

Respect also plays a vital role in creating a culture of dignity in nursing, where all individuals, regardless of their medical condition or background, are treated with compassion and empathy. In a world often starved of empathy, where patients' pain can be overshadowed by medical procedures, respect serves as a beacon of hope. By honouring the inherent dignity of each patient, we remind ourselves of our profession's ultimate purpose: to provide compassionate care that uplifts and heals.

Integrating respect into all aspects of healthcare has far-reaching implications beyond emotional validation. There is compelling evidence to suggest that respect enhances patient outcomes and satisfaction. Patients who feel respected are more likely to adhere to treatment plans, actively participate in their care, and experience greater satisfaction. Respect also strengthens patient–provider relationships, increasing trust and improving communication. These factors ultimately contribute to better health outcomes and help reduce healthcare disparities.

While respect is crucial for patients, it is equally significant for the well-being and morale of healthcare professionals. The impact of disrespectful behaviour on caregivers cannot be overstated.

Experiencing disrespect can lead to frustration, burnout, and a decline in job satisfaction. It erodes the connection between healthcare professionals and their patients, hindering effective collaboration and compromising high-quality care. Therefore, addressing and preventing disrespectful behaviour is essential for maintaining a thriving and supportive workplace environment.

Several strategies can help foster and maintain an environment of respect in healthcare settings. First, education and training programmes that emphasise respect and dignity in nursing practice can be implemented. By instilling these values early in a nurse's education, we can cultivate a generation of healthcare providers who prioritise respect as a core principle of their practice.

In addition to education, cultivating a culture of respect requires organisational policies that promote and enforce respectful behaviour. By clearly stating expectations for staff conduct and implementing consequences for violations, we create a framework within which respect becomes the norm. Organisations can also establish feedback mechanisms that provide a safe space for employees to voice concerns or report instances of disrespect, ensuring issues are addressed promptly and effectively.

Ultimately, respect is the driving force behind the evolution of nursing practice. It is an essential element that enhances patient care and uplifts the human spirit. As healthcare professionals, we must continually strive to integrate respect into every interaction, recognising its power to transform lives and shape the future of healthcare. Let us aspire to create a culture of dignity in nursing, where compassion, empathy, and respect flourish, enabling us to fulfil our most sacred duty: healing the body, mind, and soul.

Engagement: Collaboration and Teamwork in Nursing

Engagement in nursing is about being fully present and actively contributing to the success of the healthcare team. It means being a team player, collaborating with others, and using our unique skills and knowledge to provide the best possible care for our patients. As nurses, we can help others grow and succeed. By engaging in mentorship and sharing our knowledge and experiences, we empower our colleagues and inspire them to reach their full potential. Our engagement can have a ripple effect, creating a culture of learning and continuous improvement within our healthcare organisations.

Resourcefulness is another key aspect of engagement in nursing. It means being creative and innovative in finding solutions to challenges and making the most of the resources available to us. As healthcare professionals, we face complex and ever-changing situations, and by being resourceful, we can adapt and provide optimal care even in the face of adversity.

To truly understand the importance of engagement in nursing, it is crucial to discuss the benefits of collaboration and teamwork. When healthcare professionals work together towards a common goal, patient outcomes improve significantly. By leveraging each team member's knowledge, skills, and expertise, we can provide comprehensive and individualised care to our patients.

Collaboration and teamwork go beyond simply working alongside one another. They involve active participation, effective communication, and mutual respect. When we engage with our colleagues, we establish a foundation of trust and understanding, creating an environment where everyone feels valued and appreciated. This, in turn, encourages open dialogue and the exchange of ideas, leading to more informed decision-making and improved patient outcomes.

One key aspect of engagement in nursing is fostering effective teamwork. Teamwork involves recognising the strengths and weaknesses of each team member and using them to provide the best care possible. When we engage with our fellow nurses, we create a supportive network where we can learn from each other's experiences, share knowledge, and develop innovative approaches to patient care.

In a profession as demanding as nursing, resourcefulness is crucial. Engaging with our colleagues allows us to tap into a wealth of knowledge and expertise to find creative solutions to complex problems. By working collaboratively, we can combine our strengths and draw upon the team's collective intelligence. This enhances our resourcefulness and ensures that we provide the best possible care to our patients.

Engagement is also essential for our professional growth as nurses. By actively participating in collaborations and engaging with our colleagues, we expose ourselves to new perspectives, ideas, and experiences. This exposure allows us to expand our knowledge and skill sets, ultimately making us more well-rounded and adaptable nurses. Furthermore, engagement encourages continuous learning and professional development, leading to enhanced job satisfaction and a sense of fulfilment in our nursing careers.

When examining how engagement contributes to professional growth in nursing, it is important to acknowledge the role of mentorship. Engaging with experienced nurses allows us to learn from their extensive experience and wisdom. They can guide us, provide feedback, and help us navigate the challenges and complexities of our profession. By engaging with mentors, we can accelerate our professional growth and advance our nursing practice.

Furthermore, engagement in nursing promotes a positive work environment. When we actively engage with our colleagues, we help create a culture of collaboration, support, and shared responsibility. This environment fosters a sense of belonging and camaraderie, which, in turn, contributes to our overall job satisfaction. A positive work environment not only enhances teamwork and collaboration but also attracts and retains talented nurses, ensuring the delivery of high-quality patient care.

In conclusion, engagement in nursing promotes effective teamwork, resourcefulness, and professional growth. Through collaboration and teamwork, nurses can leverage their collective knowledge and skills to provide optimal patient care. Engaging with colleagues enhances our resourcefulness and fosters a positive work environment that contributes to overall job satisfaction. By actively participating in collaborations, engaging with mentors, and continually seeking opportunities for growth, we can thrive as nurses and positively impact the lives of our patients.

Excellence: Striving for the Best in Nursing

In my years of experience as a nurse, I have come to understand the importance of striving for excellence in our profession. Excellence is not merely a pursuit of perfection but a commitment to continuously improving ourselves, inspiring others, innovating, and providing the highest quality of care. In this chapter, we will explore the concept of excellence in nursing and how it empowers us to become extraordinary care providers.

Excellence is the pursuit of greatness in nursing. It is about empowering others, inspiring them to reach their full potential, and promoting innovation in healthcare. By striving for excellence, we can make a lasting impact on our patients, our colleagues, and our profession. Empowering others is a hallmark of excellent nursing practice. It involves fostering a culture of mentorship and supporting others in their professional development. By sharing our knowledge and experiences, we can inspire the next generation of nurses and create a legacy of excellence in our profession.

Healthcare innovation is essential for advancing patient care and improving outcomes. By embracing new technologies, approaches, and ideas, we can drive positive change and promote the best possible care for our patients. Excellence in nursing requires a willingness to think outside the box, challenge the status quo, and continuously seek improvement.

Excellence in nursing goes beyond the basic requirements of our profession. It involves constantly seeking ways to improve care delivery, pushing the boundaries of what is possible, and embracing innovative practices. It is about going above and beyond the call of duty, not settling for mediocrity, and always aiming for the best. When we embody excellence, we become catalysts for positive change and sources of inspiration for our colleagues and patients alike.

Imagine a nurse who consistently demonstrates exceptional clinical skills, stays updated with the latest advancements in medical knowledge, and strives to provide compassionate care to every patient. This nurse becomes a role model for others, inspiring them to reach for greatness in their practice. The pursuit of excellence sets the bar high and motivates us to learn and grow continuously, both personally and professionally. Through our commitment to excellence, we can create a ripple effect that permeates the entire healthcare team, ultimately leading to improved patient outcomes and a positive work environment.

One aspect of excellence in nursing is the ability to inspire and motivate those around us. As nurses, we are privileged to work closely with individuals who may be going through some of the most challenging times in their lives. By embodying excellence in our actions and attitudes, we can instil hope and empower our patients to take an active role in their healing journey. When patients witness our commitment to providing the highest quality of care, they are more likely to trust us, engage in their treatment plans, and experience better overall health outcomes.

Additionally, the pursuit of excellence encourages us to be innovative in our approach to care. Nursing is constantly evolving, with new technologies, research findings, and evidence-based practices emerging regularly. To provide the best possible care, we must be willing to embrace change and adapt our practices accordingly. By staying current with emerging trends and being open to new ideas, we can lead the way in implementing innovative solutions to improve patient care. Whether it is the utilisation of telehealth services, the development of interdisciplinary teams, or the integration of holistic approaches to healing, nurses who embody excellence are at the forefront of transforming healthcare delivery.

Moreover, excellence in nursing requires a commitment to self-reflection and continuous self-improvement. We must be willing to critically assess our practice, identify areas for improvement, and actively seek opportunities for professional and personal growth. This commitment to lifelong learning benefits us and enhances our ability to provide high-quality care. By regularly engaging in self-reflection, seeking feedback from colleagues, and participating in continuing education, we ensure that we are continually refining our practice and keeping pace with advancements in the field.

The CAR of Nursing

In conclusion, integrity, compassion, accountability, respect, engagement, and excellence are components of the CAR of nursing. These values form the foundation of our profession, guiding us in our interactions with patients, colleagues, and ourselves. By embodying these values in our practice, we can provide safe, compassionate, and high-quality care to those who entrust us with their well-being.

Monitoring and measuring integrity, compassion, accountability, respect, engagement, and excellence can significantly enhance our intentional living. Here are some practical methods to help you reflect on these core values daily:

Integrity: Take time each day to assess whether your actions genuinely reflect your beliefs and principles. Keeping a dedicated journal can help you document instances where you remain steadfast in your values, particularly during challenging situations. Consider reflecting on questions such as: "Did I make a decision aligned with my core beliefs today?" This practice will reinforce your commitment to living authentically.

Compassion: Make a conscious effort to track your acts of kindness, no matter their size. Each evening, ask yourself, "Did I approach those I interacted with today through the lens of empathy and understanding?" You might also set a goal to perform a specific number of thoughtful gestures each week, such as complimenting a colleague or helping a friend, making compassion a tangible aspect of your daily routine.

Accountability: Create a structured system to monitor your goals and responsibilities, using to-do lists, productivity apps, or a bullet journal. Review your progress regularly at the end of each week. When mistakes occur, practise self-reflection by acknowledging what went wrong, considering what you could have done differently, and planning actionable steps for improvement. This accountability fosters personal growth and resilience.

Respect: Reflect on how you interacted with others throughout the day. Did you genuinely listen to their concerns? Did you express appreciation for their contributions? Consider seeking constructive feedback from trusted friends, family members, or colleagues regarding your communication style and behaviour. This can provide valuable insights into how you can improve your interactions.

Engagement: Examine your level of presence and attentiveness in your daily activities, whether in conversations, work meetings, or personal projects. A gratitude log can serve as a powerful tool to help you appreciate the connections you've made. Jot down moments where you felt genuinely engaged and present, and consider how these experiences enhanced your relationships and overall well-being.

Excellence: Set specific, measurable goals in areas that resonate with you—whether in your career, personal life, or hobbies. Use a progress tracker to document your achievements and regularly assess your performance. At the end of each day, reflect on whether you gave your best effort in your pursuits. Ask yourself, "What steps did I take towards excellence today, and how can I strive for improvement tomorrow?"

To cultivate these reflections into a lasting habit, allocate 5–10 minutes every evening for journaling or self-reflection. Embodying these core values can significantly deepen your self-awareness and enrich your personal development.

Chapter 3:
The Significance of the CAR of Nursing in Holistic Care Delivery

The History of Cars

In 1886, Karl Benz unveiled the Benz Patent-Motorwagen, the world's first practical automobile. This three-wheeled vehicle, powered by a single-cylinder petrol engine, ushered in a new era of transportation. It was a revolutionary concept that captured the imagination of people across the globe.

But it was Gottlieb Daimler who truly revolutionised the automotive industry. In 1889, he introduced the Daimler Motorised Carriage, the first four-wheeled automobile. This ground-breaking invention was powered by a petrol engine and featured a lightweight design, making it a more practical mode of transportation. Daimler's innovation set the stage for the rapid development and evolution of cars in the years to come.

The early 20th century witnessed an explosion of creativity in the automotive industry. Henry Ford, a visionary entrepreneur, played an instrumental role in shaping the history of cars. In 1908, he introduced the Ford Model T, a reliable and affordable automobile that revolutionised mass production. Ford's assembly-line techniques allowed for the large-scale production of cars at a lower cost, making them accessible to a broader range of people.

With the increasing popularity of cars, their impact on transportation became undeniable. They offered convenience and autonomy never before experienced. People no longer had to rely solely on public transit or horse-drawn carriages. Cars allowed them to explore the open road and travel independently. This newfound mobility transformed the way people lived, worked, and connected.

The rise of cars also brought significant infrastructure changes. As more people embraced this mode of transportation, the need for better roads became apparent. Governments worldwide began investing in road networks, paving the way for a more interconnected society. The construction of highways, bridges, and tunnels became paramount to accommodate the increasing number of automobiles.

As cars became a common sight on the roads, their design and features continued to evolve. In the 1920s, automobile manufacturers introduced modern conveniences such as electric starters, headlights, and enclosed cabins, making driving more comfortable and safer. Technological advancements, including the invention of the automatic transmission and power steering, further enhanced the driving experience.

The impact of cars extended beyond transportation and infrastructure. The automotive industry became a cornerstone of the global economy, generating employment opportunities and driving economic growth. As car production soared, a vast network of suppliers and manufacturers emerged, creating a ripple effect that stimulated various sectors of the economy.

Cars also transformed the social fabric of society. They provided escape and adventure, allowing people to explore new places and embark on road trips. Car ownership became a symbol of status and freedom, with individuals expressing their personality and style through their choice of vehicle.

However, the rise of cars also brought challenges and concerns. The mass adoption of automobiles increased air pollution and traffic congestion in urban areas. The dependency on fossil fuels raised environmental concerns and sparked the need for more sustainable transportation alternatives. Governments and researchers began exploring electric cars and fuel-efficient engines to mitigate these issues.

Throughout the 20th and 21st centuries, cars have continued to evolve and shape the world. The introduction of hybrid and electric vehicles has brought us closer to a greener and more sustainable future. Autonomous driving technologies are revolutionising the way we think about transportation, promising increased safety and efficiency.

The CAR of Nursing

As I reflect on the incredible journey of cars, I am reminded of their transformative power. From the humble beginnings of three-wheeled contraptions to the sophisticated machines we know today, cars have undoubtedly left an indelible mark on human history. They have revolutionised transportation and become symbols of freedom, progress, and innovation. The story of cars is a testament to human ingenuity, perseverance, and our ceaseless quest for exploration and discovery.

The Birth of the Car of Nursing

My journey began with a deep dive into the annals of nursing history. I delved into the stories of Florence Nightingale, the pioneer of modern nursing, and her tireless efforts to improve patient care during the Crimean War. Nightingale's passion for nursing, relentless pursuit of knowledge, and unwavering dedication to her patients inspired me immensely.

However, her emphasis on the importance of the environment in healing caught my attention. Nightingale believed that a clean, well-ventilated, and organised space was crucial for patients' recovery. I realised that the car of nursing was an extension of this philosophy— a mobile environment designed to provide optimal care and comfort to patients wherever they may be.

I embarked on my quest to discover the birth of the car of nursing, tracing its origins back to the early 20th century. During this time, advancements in technology and transportation began to shape the world as we know it today. Once a luxury reserved for the wealthy, the automobile became more accessible to the masses, opening new possibilities.

One name that emerged prominently during my research was Lillian D. Wald, a renowned nurse and social reformer. Wald was known for her public health work and commitment to providing care to those in need. She was the first to recognise the potential of the automobile in nursing practice.

The CAR of Nursing

Wald's vision for the car of nursing took shape in the bustling streets of New York City. She envisaged a mobile healthcare unit that could bring medical services directly to patients' homes, particularly those in impoverished neighbourhoods. This concept, ahead of its time, sought to bridge the gap between healthcare access and the limitations imposed by distance and geography.

Wald's efforts were met with both admiration and scepticism. While some hailed her as a visionary, others questioned the practicality and sustainability of her idea. Undeterred, Wald sought partnerships and funding to bring her vision to life. In collaboration with the New York Visiting Nurse Service, she launched a pilot programme that deployed nurses in specially designed automobiles to deliver care to those in need.

The impact of these car-borne nurses was immediate and profound. Patients who were previously unable to access healthcare now had a lifeline, a ray of hope that illuminated the darkness of their conditions. With the car of nursing, distance was no longer a barrier to quality care. The nurses traversed the city's streets, their nursing bags filled with essential equipment and medications, ready to provide care at a moment's notice.

The success of Wald's pilot programme paved the way for further advancements in mobile nursing. Soon, other cities followed suit, adopting the concept of the car of nursing and tailoring it to their unique healthcare needs. Over the years, technological advancements further enhanced the capabilities of these mobile healthcare units.

Today, the car of nursing has evolved significantly. No longer limited to the confines of a traditional automobile, these mobile units now encompass a wide range of vehicles—from motorised vans to specialised ambulances equipped with state-of-the-art medical equipment. They bring healthcare to remote communities, disaster-stricken areas, and even war zones, offering a glimmer of hope amidst chaos and despair.

The relevance of the car of nursing in today's healthcare landscape cannot be overstated. In an era where healthcare disparities continue to plague our society, bringing care directly to the patient is more vital than ever. The car of nursing serves as a beacon of hope for marginalised, underserved, and forgotten people. It symbolises the unwavering dedication of nurses, who go above and beyond to provide care to those in need, regardless of their circumstances.

In conclusion, the birth of the car of nursing is a testament to the power of innovation and the unwavering spirit of nursing professionals. It represents the relentless pursuit of better patient outcomes and the tireless effort to break down barriers and improve access to care. As I closed this chapter, my mind was filled with newfound inspiration. Nurses around the world will all recognise a valuable yet straightforward CAR with its six components: integrity, compassion, accountability, respect, engagement, and excellent delivery. I am determined to be a part of this revolution, carry the torch of the car of nursing, and make a difference in the lives of those I will soon care for. The journey had just begun, and I was ready to embark on my own adventure in the car of nursing.

Chapter 4:
The Road Less Travelled
A Calling Discovered:

One of my earliest encounters with the world of nursing happened quite by chance. I was a teenager at the time, helping at a local community centre, when I overheard a conversation between two people that would change my life forever. The first person was a young woman, barely older than me, who spoke proudly about her chosen nursing profession. Her words were filled with an indescribable passion, and her eyes sparkled with enthusiasm as she described the fulfilment she found in caring for others. Her words captivated me, and something within me resonated deeply with the idea of making a difference in people's lives through nursing.

Inspired by this encounter, I began to explore the world of nursing and everything it had to offer. I immersed myself in books and articles, learning about the complexities of the human body and the art of compassionate care. I eagerly absorbed stories of nurses who went above and beyond their duty, touching the lives of their patients in profound ways. During this period of learning, I came across a story that struck a chord deep within my heart.

It was the story of a young boy named Saye, who had been diagnosed with a terminal illness. Saye's journey through the medical system had been long and exhausting, filled with numerous hospitalisations and painful treatments. Yet throughout it all, one nurse remained by his side, providing medical care, emotional support, and unwavering compassion. This nurse became Saye's anchor, his guiding light during his darkest moments. The impact she had on his life was immeasurable, and I could not help but imagine the difference I could make in the lives of others by following in her footsteps.

This story cemented my desire to become a nurse, and it became clear that nursing was not just a profession, but a calling. It was a calling to be a healer, a comforter, and a source of support for those in need. It was a calling to offer a shoulder to cry on, a hand to hold, and a reassuring voice in moments of uncertainty. It was a calling to stand beside people during their most vulnerable times, advocate for their needs, and provide hope in the face of adversity.

With this newfound conviction, I embarked on the path towards nursing. I enrolled in nursing studies, beginning with Certificate III in Aged Care, progressing through a Diploma of Nursing, and eventually completing a Bachelor of Nursing. I was ready to learn the practical skills and knowledge needed to fulfil my calling. Yet it was not only classroom learning that shaped me; it was my clinical experiences that truly brought everything to life.

During my clinical placements, I witnessed the daily realities of nursing. I saw the joy on a mother's face as she held her newborn for the first time, and I felt the weight of grief as I held the hand of a dying patient in their final moments. These experiences were both humbling and empowering, reminding me of the profound impact nurses have on the lives of their patients.

Each story and every encounter with patients and their families only strengthened my passion. It was in those moments of genuine connection, when the boundaries of professionalism softened and we became fellow humans navigating illness and healing together, that I felt the true depth of my calling. I realised that nursing was not just a job; it was a privilege and an honour to be entrusted with the care of others during their most vulnerable moments.

In the darkest of times, nurses shine a light within the tunnel, offering solace, comfort, and care. They stand beside their patients, providing guidance and support on the path towards better health. They make a difference, not only in individual lives, but in the wider world.

As I reflect on my journey towards discovering my true calling in nursing, I am filled with gratitude. I am grateful for the chance encounter that sparked the flame within me, grateful for the stories that inspired me, and grateful for the opportunity to make a difference in the lives of others. I know that my path as a nurse will not always be easy, but the reward of knowing that I have touched a life, provided comfort, or instilled hope will outweigh any challenges along the way.

Nursing is not just a career; it is a way of life. It is a calling that demands compassion, dedication, and a commitment to serving others. For me, it is the most rewarding and fulfilling calling I could have ever discovered.

Navigating the Unknown:

As I stepped into the world of nursing, I felt as though I had boarded a ship bound for a wild and unpredictable voyage. Waves of uncertainty crashed against the bow, threatening to overwhelm my novice heart. This was a journey that required learning to navigate the unknown, letting go of the safety of textbooks and embracing the reality of the hospital ward.

Day one was an avalanche of emotions. My hands trembled as I slid the key card into the door, revealing the world of patient care that awaited me. The sterile scent filled my senses, mingling with the anxiety swirling inside me. I took a deep breath, steadying myself to face the challenges ahead.

The first challenge I encountered was the infamous art of bedpans. In nursing education, you learn the theory behind personal care, but nothing fully prepares you for the practical reality. It was a delicate balance of vulnerability and respect as I learned to navigate this intimate aspect of patient care. Each patient had their own preferences, and I had to find the balance between efficiency and empathy.

With time and experience, I refined my skills. I learned subtle techniques to make the process less confronting, ensuring patients felt both dignity and comfort. Helping someone feel at ease during their most vulnerable moments became a reward in itself. I realised that despite its challenges, nursing allowed me to be a small but meaningful part of someone's healing journey.

However, bedpans were only the beginning. As I delved deeper into nursing, I encountered a wide range of patients, each with unique needs and expectations. Managing these demands became an art, requiring patience, organisation, and a fair amount of multitasking.

Every shift brought new patients with varied conditions, each requiring care tailored to their situation. There were elderly patients with frail bodies whose gentle manner reminded me of the importance of tenderness. There were also more challenging cases, where I had to rely on persuasion and negotiation to encourage adherence to treatment plans.

I quickly learned that nursing was not only about caring for the body, but also about healing the spirit. A smile or a reassuring touch could ease pain and fear in ways that medication alone could not. These small moments of connection strengthened my resolve to continue in this demanding profession.

As days turned into weeks, and weeks into months and years, I began to find my footing amid the unknown. The tears that once flowed from self-doubt were gradually replaced by the support and camaraderie of fellow nurses, who understood the struggle and offered encouragement without judgement. We became a close-knit group, navigating the challenges of nursing together.

The laughter that filled the break room during our short respite from the chaos became my lifeline. We shared stories of triumphs and mishaps, finding solace in each other's experiences. There was a unique understanding among us, as we all knew what it felt like to juggle endless demands and still find the strength to keep going.

Navigating the unknown didn't just involve mastering the practical aspects of nursing; it also required a deep understanding of human nature. Every patient had a story, hidden beneath the layers of pain and illness. To truly navigate their unknown, I had to unravel their narratives, piece by piece, like a detective piecing together a puzzle.

Listening became an essential skill, allowing me to decode the language of their symptoms and fears. The mumbled complaints, the nervous laughter, the silent tears – each carried a message, waiting to be understood. Through my presence, I became the bridge that connected their fears to the torch of hope.

Some moments were tough, like when we couldn't save a life despite our best efforts. It was during those times that my unwavering determination faced its greatest test. I was brought to the precipice of despair, tempted to believe that the unknown was too dark to navigate. But it was in those moments of hardship that I realized the strength that resided within me.

I rose from doubt with a renewed determination to make a difference, even when the outcome was not what I had hoped for. Each loss became a reminder that nursing is a balance of joy and heartbreak, and that the privilege of walking alongside someone on their journey makes it worthwhile.

As I reflect on the early years of my nursing career, I am struck by how much I have grown. I have travelled through uncharted waters, embracing the unknown with humility and resilience. These trials have shaped me, moulding me into a clinical nurse capable of remaining compassionate amid chaos.

Navigating the unknown is not about having all the answers. It is about trusting the journey and trusting yourself. It means accepting uncertainty while knowing you have the strength to face whatever lies ahead. Nursing, with all its challenges and rewards, has taught me to navigate the unknown with grace and steadfast determination.

Chapter 5:
Healing Hearts, One Beat at a Time
A Symphony of Compassion:

In nursing, compassion is not merely a soft skill, but a symphony that guides the healing process. It is the harmony that connects patient and nurse on an emotional level, creating trust and comfort. This symphony begins with gentle notes of understanding, as the nurse takes time to listen and truly understand a patient's concerns and fears.

One particular memory stands out, a moment of connection that extended beyond the walls of the hospital room. I remember Mrs Johnson, a frail elderly woman who had recently undergone a complex surgery. She was visibly anxious, her hands trembling as she struggled to express her fears. I sat beside her, gently holding her hand and reassuring her that she was not alone on this journey. This simple act of presence and support appeared to calm her, as though the symphony of compassion had wrapped her in a soothing embrace.

The transformative power of compassion was evident as I continued to care for Mrs. Johnson. I would visit her daily, not only to fulfill my professional duties but also to provide emotional support. We would engage in conversations that ranged from memories of her youth to her concerns about the future. I learned about her family, her dreams, and her fears. Through these moments of connection, a bond was formed, and Mrs. Johnson felt seen and valued as an individual rather than just another patient.

Compassion, like music, can transcend language barriers. This became evident in my interactions with Mr Rodriguez, a non English speaking patient who had suffered a stroke. Communication could easily have been difficult, with limited translation resources available. Yet I learned that compassion has a universal language that extends beyond words. I would sit by his bedside, hold his hand, and offer a reassuring presence. By observing his non verbal cues and responding with care, a meaningful connection was formed. The symphony of compassion was not expressed through speech, but through presence, understanding, and reassurance.

Compassion also extends beyond patients to include their loved ones. The symphony of compassion can ease the fears and anxieties of family members, offering comfort during moments of uncertainty. I recall a situation where a young child was admitted to the emergency department following a serious accident. The parents were distraught, their faces marked by fear and distress. While caring for their child, I made a deliberate effort to support them emotionally as well. I sat with them, listened to their concerns, and offered reassurance. Together, we navigated the overwhelming uncertainty, finding comfort through shared compassion.

In today's fast paced healthcare environment, it is easy to become overwhelmed by workload and pressure. Yet it is often the small, everyday acts of kindness that make the greatest difference. A smile, a gentle touch, or simply listening can alter the course of a patient's experience. These moments of compassion create a safe space where vulnerability can be expressed and understood.

The power of compassion is not limited to patients alone; it also has a profound effect on nurses. Reflecting on my own experiences, I have seen how compassionate care can ease the emotional weight of the profession. Through these acts, nurses find purpose and resilience, drawing strength to continue caring for others even during challenging times.

The symphony of compassion is not a single performance, but an ongoing journey. It requires nurses to continually strive for empathy and remain attentive to the needs of those in their care. This symphony is created in partnership with patients, families, and the wider healthcare team. Its influence extends beyond individual encounters, shaping the overall healthcare experience.

As we move forward, we must remember the impact that even the smallest gestures of compassion can have. Let us embrace the symphony woven through our interactions, recognising the power of empathy and kindness. Together, we can foster a healing environment where patients find comfort, reassurance, and hope during their most vulnerable moments.

When Words Fail, Music Speaks:

I began to play a familiar tune, one that had been a constant presence in her life for decades. The gentle melody of her favourite song filled the room, surrounding us in warmth and comfort. I watched as Mrs Johnson's rigid posture softened, her tense muscles gradually relaxing. The corners of her mouth lifted slightly, as though a cherished memory had resurfaced.

Music has long been recognised as a universal language, capable of reaching deep within us and evoking emotions that words cannot express. In nursing, its healing potential has become increasingly evident, offering comfort that transcends verbal communication.

Throughout my nursing career, I have witnessed countless moments where music served as a bridge, reconnecting patients with their past, easing anxiety, and providing relief from pain and uncertainty. In my current role within the rehabilitation unit, many patients choose to listen to their favourite music while working towards their recovery goals.

One memory remains particularly vivid. It was a typical night on the paediatric ward, filled with the cries of frightened children. I entered the room of a young girl named Comba, who was scheduled for a delicate surgical procedure the following day. Anxiety radiated from her, overwhelming and palpable.

I sat down beside her, gently strumming the chords like I was playing a guitar, and began to sing a lullaby. As my voice filled the room, the tension melted away from Comba's face, and her rapid breathing slowed. Her wide eyes, once filled with panic, now grew heavy with fatigue. The melody seemed to transport her to a place far away from the sterile hospital environment, cradling her in a cocoon of safety and peace.

In geriatric care, I have also seen the remarkable impact of music. Dementia, with its devastating effects on memory and cognition, often leaves older adults feeling isolated. Yet when a familiar song fills the room, it can transport them back to a time of clarity and connection.

One afternoon, I sat with Mr John, a resident in a memory care facility. Music had once been central to his life, his fingers moving effortlessly across piano keys. Dementia had taken much from him, leaving confusion and frustration in its wake. As his favourite piece played, his face lit up with recognition. Though his speech was fragmented, his hands began to move instinctively, mimicking the motions of playing the piano. His fingers danced through the air, telling a story shaped by a lifetime of music and memories.

Research has provided ample evidence to support the therapeutic effects of music in healthcare settings. Studies have shown that music can decrease stress hormones, lower blood pressure, and elevate mood. It can awaken dormant memories, even in patients with advanced dementia, reminding them of moments of joy and celebration.

But beyond the scientific realm, music has an intangible power that defies explanation. It reaches into the depths of our beings, addressing the pain and longing that words alone cannot soothe. It allows us to connect on a level that transcends language, culture, and even time.

In my years as a nurse, I have come to realize that the healing power of music is not limited to the patient alone. It acts as a conduit, carrying us through the darkest moments of our profession, igniting hope and reminding us why we chose this path.

As I reflect on the countless moments when music has comforted patients, I am reminded of the incredible privilege I have as a nurse. Witnessing the transformation that occurs when words fail and music steps in to fill the void is a gift that cannot be quantified.

So, as I continue my journey in the field of nursing, I carry with me the knowledge that in times of despair and incomprehension, when words fall short, there is always music to speak to the souls of those in need. And in that harmonious language, we find solace, connection, and the beauty of healing.

Chapter 6:
Navigation of compassion care

Culturally competent in nursing.

As I tread upon the path of nursing, I have come to realize that the fundamental aspect of compassionate care lies in the ability to recognise, respect, and embrace the rich diversity of humanity. Every person encountered within the healthcare setting brings with them a unique set of cultural beliefs, values, and practices that influence how they perceive health, illness, and wellbeing. This understanding has led me to explore cultural competence in depth, as I firmly believe it is an essential skill for every nurse.

Within the pages of *The CAR of Nursing*, I aim to highlight the importance of cultural competence in delivering truly compassionate care. Drawing on experiences that have shaped my professional journey, I explore the significant impact cultural competence has on patient outcomes, the importance of overcoming language and communication barriers, its role in addressing healthcare disparities, and the value of training and education in strengthening cultural competence among nursing professionals.

1: The Impact of Cultural Competence on Patient Outcomes

As I reflect on my experiences, countless moments reinforce the importance of cultural competence in improving patient outcomes. Research consistently suggests that when healthcare providers demonstrate cultural competence, patients are more likely to experience positive health outcomes. This connection exists for several reasons. When nurses understand and respect diverse cultural beliefs, values, and practices, they are better positioned to establish trust and empathy with their patients. This trust supports open and effective communication, enabling a clearer understanding of patients' symptoms, concerns, and expectations. When patients feel heard, respected, and understood, they are more likely to participate actively in their care, adhere to treatment plans, and ultimately achieve better health outcomes.

2: Overcoming Language and Communication Barriers

At the core of cultural competence is the ability to overcome language and communication barriers. As nurses, we have a responsibility to bridge the gaps created by linguistic diversity and ensure that communication remains central to compassionate care. When patients and providers lack a shared language, it can lead to misunderstandings, misdiagnoses, and a marked decline in the quality of care delivered. In this chapter, I will explore the strategies and best practices that have proven effective in communicating with patients from diverse cultural backgrounds, particularly those with limited English proficiency. By harnessing the power of interpretation services, employing bilingual staff, and utilizing culturally sensitive communication tools, nurses can foster a bond of understanding that goes beyond language barriers.

To communicate effectively with patients who have limited English proficiency, nurses can adopt a range of thoughtful strategies to ensure patients feel supported and understood:

Use professional interpreters: Wherever possible, certified medical interpreters should be used. These professionals are trained in medical terminology, ethical standards, and accurate translation, reducing the risk of miscommunication that may arise when relying on family members or friends as interpreters.

1. *Tips when using* a professional interpreter. Brief the interpreter on the context and key points of the conversation. Speak *directly to the patient* (not *the interpreter*) to maintain a personal connection. Allow the interpreter to pause *and* relay information accurately.

2. **2. Leverage Technology**: The use of translation apps and devices can be beneficial; however, it is essential to assess their reliability, particularly regarding medical terminology. Some apps may not accurately translate complex medical language, which could lead to potentially harmful miscommunication. Consider using

reputable translation services specifically designed for healthcare settings.

3. **3. Provide Written Materials:** Offering educational **materials** translated into the patient's preferred language can significantly aid understanding. These materials should include straightforward language and be accompanied by visual aids, such as diagrams or infographics, to further clarify complex concepts and instructions.

4. **4. Learn Key Phrases:** Familiarizing oneself with essential **phrases** in the patient's language can significantly ease communication. This effort demonstrates an investment in the patient's comfort and builds rapport, making them feel more at ease in a healthcare setting.

5. **5. Speak Clearly and Slowly:** Nurses should use simple language and avoid technical jargon when communicating. Speaking slowly and enunciating gives patients the time to process information, which is particularly important when grappling with language barriers.

6. **6. Use Nonverbal Communication**: Emphasizing nonverbal cues—gestures, facial expressions, and visual aids—can transcend language barriers. These forms of communication can effectively convey meaning and emotional context, helping to enhance understanding and comfort.

7. **7. Collaborate with Cultural Brokers**: Engaging with **cultural brokers**—individuals with deep knowledge of the patient's cultural background—can provide invaluable insights. These professionals can facilitate more nuanced communication and help navigate cultural sensitivities affecting healthcare interactions.

8. **8. Build** Trust: Establishing a trusting relationship requires displaying empathy, patience, and respect for cultural differences. Taking the time to understand patients' backgrounds and feelings fosters a supportive environment, which can lead to improved communication and patient satisfaction.

By applying these approaches, healthcare providers can improve understanding, increase patient satisfaction, and achieve better health outcomes for patients with limited English proficiency.

3: Addressing Healthcare Disparities

Cultural competence plays a vital role in reducing healthcare disparities that continue to affect many cultural and ethnic groups. Unfortunately, access to healthcare is not equal for all, and disparities in care quality and health outcomes are often rooted in cultural bias and structural inequality. In this chapter, I explore how cultural competence enables nurses to identify and address these inequities. By recognising social determinants of health and acknowledging the influence of culture, nurses can advocate for fair and inclusive healthcare. Through culturally sensitive assessments, personalised care plans, and inclusive policies, nursing professionals can contribute to a more just and compassionate healthcare system.

4: Training and Education in Cultural Competence

Developing cultural competence within nursing requires a strong foundation in education and training. These experiences provide the knowledge, skills, and attitudes needed to work effectively within diverse healthcare environments. In the following chapter, I examine the effectiveness of various training programs and educational initiatives aimed at enhancing cultural competence among nurses. By evaluating these approaches, we can identify the most effective strategies and promote a culture of ongoing learning and professional growth.

As I continue this exploration into cultural competence, I invite you to engage with the diverse stories presented throughout *The CAR of Nursing*. Together, we can navigate the broad landscape of human diversity and uncover the insights held within culture. Through shared understanding, I believe we can help shape a future of compassionate care that is inclusive, respectful, and responsive to all.

5: Palliative and End-of-life Care

As a nurse, I have witnessed the profound impact of palliative and end-of-life care on patients and their families. These delicate situations demand extraordinary compassion, skill, and understanding. Throughout my career, I have encountered numerous challenges and considerations in providing this specialised form of care. In this chapter, we will explore the intricacies of palliative and end-of-life care, delving into the emotional, ethical, and practical dilemmas accompanying these profound moments.

To truly comprehend the complexities of palliative and end-of-life care, it is necessary to understand its historical roots. As I delve into the pages of history, I am struck by the gradual evolution of societies' approach towards death. In previous eras, death was often shrouded in secrecy and silence, and the dying were often isolated from their loved ones. I experienced this at age 5 when my father was seriously sick or dying. My little sisters and I were taken away from home to my uncle house, which is just few blocks away. We were not allowed to go back home until after two days of his burial. The advent of palliative care in the 20th century marked a significant shift, as it embraced the concept of relieving suffering and enhancing quality of life for those approaching the end of their journey.

It is both our duty and an innate human responsibility to provide compassionate care during these final moments. However, the challenges we encounter in this endeavour can be overwhelming. One such challenge lies in managing the various physical symptoms experienced by patients in palliative and end-of-life care. Pain, nausea, and shortness of breath are just a few of the distressing symptoms that necessitate our prompt attention and expertise. We must constantly assess, reassess, and adjust the medication regimens and comfort measures to alleviate suffering. This meticulous balancing act requires not only a deep understanding of pharmacology but also the ability to truly listen to patients, as their communication may be impaired due to their condition.

But the challenges faced in palliative and end-of-life care extend far beyond the realm of physical symptoms. Among the most profound challenges is the emotional toll it takes on both patients and healthcare providers. Witnessing the decline of a patient we have come to know and care for can be emotionally gruelling. We must learn to navigate our own emotions while remaining steadfast in our commitment to providing compassionate care. It is imperative to recognize the importance of self-care and to seek support from our teams, as the journey through palliative and end-of-life care can be an arduous one.

Another challenge that arises involves the ethical considerations that accompany these situations. Each person approaches end of life differently, and respecting their autonomy and informed choices is paramount. As healthcare providers, we must remain mindful of cultural and religious preferences, personal beliefs, and legal responsibilities. Ethical dilemmas may include discussions about withholding or withdrawing life sustaining treatments, engaging in advance care planning, or navigating complex family dynamics. In these moments, our moral judgement is tested, and we must respond with empathy, sensitivity, and a commitment to delivering the best possible care for all involved.

Attention to family dynamics and the psychosocial impact of end of life care on loved ones is another crucial aspect. Grief and loss are powerful emotions, and it is our responsibility to support families as they move through this difficult journey. Creating an environment that encourages open communication and active listening can offer vital emotional support during these challenging times. Providing resources and education that help families understand the stages of grief, from denial and anger through to acceptance and peace, is essential in walking this tender path together.

Amid these challenges, it is important to remember that palliative and end of life care extends beyond physical, emotional, and ethical considerations. It is about fostering moments of connection, compassion, and dignity. It is about preserving quality of life until the final breath. Delivering compassionate care requires a shift in professional perspective, seeing the patient as a whole person rather than a set of symptoms or a diagnosis. We must seek to understand their hopes, fears, and wishes, and honour their individuality throughout their end of life journey.

In conclusion, palliative and end of life care is a complex and deeply meaningful aspect of nursing practice. The challenges we face in providing compassionate care during these sensitive times are significant. From managing physical symptoms and witnessing emotional distress, to addressing ethical dilemmas and supporting families, every aspect of our professional and personal selves is tested. Yet we are continually reminded of the privilege it is to accompany patients and their loved ones on such an intimate and sacred journey. By embracing this complexity and committing to a holistic approach, we ensure that the CAR of nursing shines brightest in moments of darkness, offering comfort, care, and compassion until the end.

Chapter 7:
Highlighting the Significance of Trauma Informed Care in Promoting Compassionate Healing:

As a clinical nurse with eight years of experience working in a rehabilitation unit, I often reflect on the importance of trauma informed care in nursing. I am reminded of the many stories shared by patients who have endured deep and lasting trauma. Their pain is evident in tear filled eyes and trembling voices. In these moments, I recognise the true significance of trauma informed care and its capacity to change lives.

Trauma informed care is not a passing concept or a trend in nursing. It represents a fundamental shift in how we approach the physical, emotional, and psychological wellbeing of our patients. It acknowledges that trauma can shape every aspect of a person's life and that healing begins with recognising and addressing its impact.

In the past, healthcare professionals may have unintentionally intensified the suffering of trauma survivors. Care was sometimes delivered in a detached and clinical manner, lacking empathy and understanding. Today, we must do better. As nurses, we are called to embrace trauma informed care as a core principle of our practice.

To truly comprehend the significance of trauma-informed care, we must first recognize the prevalence of trauma in our society. Research shows that trauma affects individuals from all walks of life, regardless of age, gender, or social status. Whether it be childhood abuse, witnessing violence, or surviving a natural disaster, trauma leaves an indelible mark on the human psyche.

Through my journey as a nurse, I have come to understand the far-reaching effects of trauma. It infiltrates every aspect of a person's life, shaping their thoughts, behaviours, and relationships. Many trauma survivors live in a perpetual state of hypervigilance, constantly on edge and anticipating further harm. They often exhibit symptoms of anxiety, depression, and post-traumatic stress disorder (PTSD), which can manifest as physical illnesses or manifest in self-destructive behaviours.

By incorporating trauma-informed care into the framework of nursing practice, we can create an environment where individuals feel safe, valued, and empowered to embark on the path to healing. It begins with a radical shift in our mindset, acknowledging that their past does not define those who have experienced trauma but are capable of growth and resilience.

A key component of trauma informed care is the development of a safe and supportive therapeutic relationship. Nurses must listen actively, allowing patients to share their experiences without judgement or interruption. This validation can help restore dignity and self-worth to individuals who have felt unseen or powerless.

In addition to providing a safe space for expression, trauma-informed care necessitates a deep understanding of the neurobiological impact of trauma. Research has shown that trauma can alter brain development, leading to modifications in the areas responsible for emotional regulation and cognitive functioning. This knowledge is crucial in tailoring our nursing interventions to address the specific needs of trauma survivors.

A trauma-informed approach also emphasizes the importance of choice and autonomy. Trauma survivors have often experienced a loss of control over their own lives, feeling overwhelmed by the circumstances that brought them to our care. By empowering them to make decisions about their treatment and involving them in the development of their care plan, we can help restore a sense of agency that has been taken away from them.

But trauma-informed care is not just about individual interactions; it permeates every aspect of healthcare systems. It calls for a multidisciplinary approach, where professionals from various disciplines collaborate to provide holistic care. This approach ensures continuity of care and prevents traumatization.

Furthermore, trauma-informed care extends beyond the walls of the healthcare setting. It necessitates a shift in society's perceptions and attitudes towards trauma, eradicates the stigma surrounding mental health, and promotes compassion and understanding. It is a collective effort to create a world where every trauma survivor is met with empathy and support, rather than judgment and isolation.

As nurses, we are in a unique position to champion trauma-informed care. We hold the power to be agents of change, to transform the healthcare landscape into one that fosters healing, growth, and resilience. It may not always be easy; trauma is complex, and its impact far-reaching. But if we approach our practice with an unwavering commitment to trauma-informed care, we have the power to ignite hope in the hearts of those who have lost their way.

The significance of trauma-informed care lies not only in its potential to promote individual healing but also in its power to reshape the face of healthcare as we know it. It is a paradigm shift, a call to action, and a testament to the transformative impact nurses can have on the lives of their patients. Let us rise to the occasion, embracing trauma-informed care as the cornerstone of compassionate healing. Together, we can create a future where trauma survivors are no longer defined by their pain but are empowered by their resilience.

Care for Vulnerable Populations

Throughout my nursing career, I have encountered many situations where providing compassionate care to vulnerable populations presented distinct challenges. One such experience involved an elderly patient, Mrs Dahn, aged seventy. She was admitted to hospital with multiple chronic conditions and limited mobility, creating a range of complexities in her care.

Mrs Dahn experienced significant feelings of isolation and loneliness. Her limited mobility confined her mostly to her room, reducing opportunities for interaction with others. It became essential for me to provide not only medical care but emotional support as well. Spending additional time with her, engaging in conversation, and showing genuine interest in her life helped reduce her sense of isolation. By offering a listening ear and consistent presence, I was able to bring comfort amid her physical discomfort.

She also faced difficulties communicating her needs clearly. Age related cognitive decline made it challenging to assess her symptoms accurately. This required a patient and attentive approach, using both verbal and nonverbal communication strategies. Careful observation, simplified language, and attentive listening helped me better understand her needs and deliver appropriate care.

Financial hardship further complicated Mrs Dahn's situation, as she struggled to afford essential medications and medical supplies. In response, I took on an advocacy role, connecting her with social services and exploring available supports. Through collaboration with social workers and case managers, we secured financial assistance and developed a plan to ensure she had access to the medications and supplies required for her ongoing care.

In addition to these challenges, vulnerable populations often face social determinants of health that significantly impact their wellbeing. Factors such as poverty, access to healthcare, and education play a crucial role in overall health outcomes. Understanding and addressing these determinants is essential in providing compassionate and effective care to these populations.

For instance, when caring for people experiencing homelessness, it is vital to recognise the barriers they face beyond their immediate healthcare needs. Many lack stable housing, access to nutritious food, and appropriate hygiene facilities, all of which can greatly affect their overall health and wellbeing. As a nurse, I have found it necessary to collaborate with community organisations and social services to deliver holistic care that addresses these social determinants. By connecting individuals with services that provide shelter, food, and ongoing support, we can help establish a more stable foundation from which they can improve their health and wellbeing.

Similarly, when caring for children from vulnerable populations, such as those in foster care or living in low-income communities, it is important to consider the influence of their environment on their health. Children in these situations often experience adversity, trauma, and limited access to healthcare and education. As a nurse, I have found it essential to advocate for these children to ensure they receive the resources and support necessary for healthy development. By working collaboratively with child protection services, educators, and community organisations, we can provide comprehensive care that addresses their physical, emotional, and educational needs.

The challenges of providing compassionate care to vulnerable populations are many, but with the right mindset and approach, we can make a meaningful difference in their lives. This requires a deep sense of empathy for their unique circumstances, a commitment to advocating for their needs, and resilience in the face of systemic barriers. As nurses, we have the capacity to be agents of change, to bridge gaps in healthcare, and to provide care that extends beyond surface-level interventions.

In conclusion, caring for vulnerable populations is a fundamental aspect of nursing practice. It requires a thorough understanding of the challenges these individuals face and the ability to approach their care with compassion and empathy. By recognising the social determinants of health, advocating for their needs, and collaborating with community resources, we can provide care that addresses both immediate medical concerns and the underlying factors affecting their wellbeing. The CAR of nursing, with its emphasis on compassion, advocacy, and resilience, is especially vital when caring for vulnerable populations. Through our collective efforts, we have the power to make a genuine difference and contribute to a more equitable healthcare system.

Self-Compassion in Nursing:

As nurses, our ability to provide compassionate care to others is closely linked to our understanding and practice of self-compassion. In this chapter, we explore the concept of self-compassion and its importance in nursing. By recognising its value, we can enhance our own wellbeing, improve patient outcomes, and foster a culture of empathy and understanding within healthcare settings.

Defining Self-Compassion:

Self-compassion is often misunderstood as self-pity or self-indulgence, but it is far removed from these ideas. It involves treating ourselves with the same kindness, warmth, and understanding that we would offer a close friend during times of difficulty. Dr Kristin Neff, a leading researcher in this field, defines self-compassion as comprising three key elements: self-kindness, common humanity, and mindfulness.

Self-Kindness:

Practising self-kindness means offering ourselves care and support during times of stress, rather than engaging in harsh self-criticism. As nurses, we are often taught that self-sacrifice is a virtue. While commitment to our profession is essential, neglecting our own wellbeing can undermine our capacity to provide compassionate care. By embracing self-kindness, we acknowledge our own emotional needs, which in turn enables us to connect more deeply with our patients.

Common Humanity:

Recognising our common humanity is a vital aspect of self-compassion. It reminds us that we are not alone in our struggles, even when our experiences feel isolating. Nurses regularly witness the suffering of others, and this exposure can have a significant emotional impact. By understanding that difficulty and suffering are shared human experiences, we can develop empathy not only for our patients but also for ourselves.

Mindfulness:

Mindfulness involves being present in the moment without judgment. In the context of self-compassion, it means acknowledging and accepting our thoughts and emotions, whether positive or negative, without becoming overwhelmed by them. Nursing often involves high-pressure situations, and it can be easy to become consumed by stress or self-judgment. By practising mindfulness, we can observe our internal experiences with greater balance, allowing us to respond with clarity and compassion.

Importance of Self-Compassion in Nursing:

Self-compassion is not merely a personal quality; it offers substantial benefits for both nurses and their patients. Research indicates that nurses who practise self-compassion experience lower levels of burnout, greater job satisfaction, and improved overall wellbeing. When we prioritise our own care, we are better positioned to deliver high-quality patient care.

Enhanced Emotional Resilience:

Nursing is a demanding profession that exposes us to the emotional challenges faced by our patients. Without self-compassion, we may become emotionally exhausted and eventually lose our sense of empathy. By fostering self-compassion, however, we can develop emotional resilience - the ability to adapt and cope with the stresses of our profession while continuing to provide compassionate care.

Improved Patient Outcomes:

When nurses practice self-compassion, it positively impacts patient outcomes. Research has shown that nurses who are more self-compassionate have higher levels of empathy and are better able to connect with their patients on a deeper level. This connection promotes trust and fosters a more therapeutic nurse-patient relationship, ultimately leading to improved health outcomes and patient satisfaction.

Creating a Culture of Compassion:

To create a culture of compassion within healthcare settings, it is essential for nurses to embody self-compassion. When we practice self-compassion, we become role models for our colleagues and inspire others to prioritize their own well-being. By encouraging self-compassion in the workplace, we can foster a supportive and nurturing environment that values empathy and compassionate care.

Conclusion:

Self-compassion is not a luxury; it is a necessity for nurses. By exploring the concept of self-compassion and understanding its importance in our profession, we can cultivate a deep sense of empathy, enhance patient care, and improve our own well-being. As nurses, our ability to provide compassionate care begins with being compassionate to ourselves. Through self-kindness, an understanding of our common humanity, and mindfulness, we can pave the way towards a brighter and more compassionate future in nursing.

By embodying self-compassion, we become catalysts for positive change, not only within our profession but also within ourselves. Let us embark on this journey of self-discovery and self-care, for in doing so, we unlock the true potential of compassionate nursing.

Chapter 8:
The Wheels of Compassion

Active Listening

Active listening is an essential skill that forms the foundation of my communication with patients and clients. It goes beyond simply hearing their words and extends to understanding their emotions, concerns, and needs. Through active listening, we establish a meaningful connection with our patients, positively influencing their overall care and wellbeing.

Building Trust and Rapport:

When we engage in active listening, it creates the conditions for trust to develop between us and our patients. Open and honest communication is vital in building a therapeutic relationship, as it fosters a sense of comfort and safety. Patients who feel heard and understood are more likely to share vital information about their health, leading to accurate assessments and diagnoses.

Moreover, active listening allows us to acknowledge our patients' emotions and perspectives. By validating their feelings and concerns, we create a supportive environment that reassures them and instils a sense of belonging and empathy. This ultimately leads to increased patient satisfaction and strengthens the relationship between patient and nurse.

Enhancing Patient Satisfaction and Experience:

Active listening plays a key role in improving patient satisfaction and their overall experience within the healthcare system. Patients often feel anxious, vulnerable, and overwhelmed by a complex and unfamiliar environment. When they perceive that their healthcare providers are genuinely listening, it creates a sense of importance and respect.

Active listening enables us to respond to patients' needs promptly and effectively, helping them feel valued and acknowledged. By actively involving patients in the decision-making process, we empower them to take ownership of their care, resulting in a greater sense of control and autonomy. This personalised approach enhances the patient experience, as they feel engaged in their treatment plan, increasing overall satisfaction.

Improving Patient Outcomes and Treatment Adherence:

The impact of active listening on patient outcomes cannot be underestimated. When patients trust that their concerns are genuinely heard, they are more likely to follow treatment plans and adhere to medication regimens. Active listening helps us identify barriers to adherence, such as concerns about side effects, financial limitations, or personal beliefs.

Additionally, through active listening, we gain a deeper understanding of our patient's health literacy and their understanding of their condition. This knowledge allows us to tailor our explanations and education to their level of comprehension, promoting better self-management skills. With improved comprehension and adherence, patient outcomes are enhanced, resulting in improved health and well-being.

Reducing Medical Errors and Ensuring Patient Safety:

Active listening is not only vital for patient satisfaction and outcomes, but also plays an important role in ensuring patient safety and reducing medical errors. The ability to listen carefully to patients' concerns and questions allows us to identify potential errors or misunderstandings in their care plans.

By actively listening, we are better positioned to identify critical information, such as allergies or previous adverse reactions to medications, which can significantly affect patient safety. In addition, patients may share important details about their medical history or previous investigations that may have been missed in electronic health records.

Through active listening, we also support effective handovers and communication within the healthcare team, ensuring that essential information is accurately shared with relevant providers. This clear and consistent communication reduces the risk of errors and enhances patient safety.

Strategies and Techniques for Developing Active Listening Skills:

Becoming an active listener requires ongoing practice and refinement of communication skills. While each nurse's approach may vary, several effective strategies can be used to develop active listening skills.

Firstly, it is crucial to create a conducive environment for active listening. This includes finding a quiet and private space to engage in open and focused conversation. Minimizing distractions, such as turning off unnecessary electronic devices or closing doors, allows for better concentration and attentiveness.

Non-verbal communication must not be overlooked when engaging in active listening. Maintaining good eye contact and using affirmative nodding or other encouraging gestures demonstrates interest and involvement. It is important to keep an open posture, leaning slightly towards the patient to demonstrate attentiveness and create a sense of approachability. These non-verbal cues enhance the patient's perception of being actively listened to.

As a nurse and life coach, patience and allowing patients and clients sufficient time to express their thoughts and concerns fully are essential. Interrupting or rushing conversations can hinder effective communication and weaken trust. Silence and pauses should be accepted, as they allow patients the space to gather their thoughts and share their experiences without pressure.

Another valuable technique in active listening is paraphrasing or summarising what the patient has shared. This demonstrates that their words have been heard and understood. By restating their concerns or questions, patients are encouraged to expand or clarify, supporting a deeper understanding of their needs. This technique, among others, works particularly well for me, as English is my second language.

Reflective listening is another effective method that can be used in active listening. By reflecting the emotions expressed by the patient, we validate their experience and encourage them to explore their concerns further. This may be as simple as saying, "It sounds like you're feeling overwhelmed by this situation. Can you tell me more about what you're going through?"

Active listening also involves being mindful of non-verbal cues, such as body language, tone of voice, and facial expressions. Paying attention to changes in these cues helps us to gauge the patient's emotional state and level of engagement. Responding empathetically to their emotions, such as sadness or fear, conveys validation and understanding. For instance, saying, "I can see that this news is difficult for you. I'm here to support you through this journey," can provide immense comfort to patients.

In conclusion, active listening is a skill that has a profound impact on patient care. By focusing wholeheartedly on patients and demonstrating empathy, nurses can build trust, enhance patient experience and satisfaction, improve adherence to treatment plans, reduce medical errors, and ultimately ensure the safety and well-being of their patients. Through the strategies and techniques outlined, nurses can develop and refine their active listening skills, transforming the trajectory of patient care.

Empathetic Presence:

As I continue my journey through writing the CAR of nursing, I have come to recognise the importance of being present and empathetic in my profession. Through these qualities, I can connect with my patients on a deeper and more meaningful level, offering the care and support they need during vulnerable moments. In this chapter, I explore how presence and empathy enhance the care of nursing, enabling us to better understand and address the emotional and psychological needs of our patients.

To fully understand the significance of empathetic presence in nursing, it is essential to consider its historical context. Nursing has evolved over the years from a primarily task-oriented profession to one that recognizes the crucial role of emotional and psychological support in patient care. In the early days of nursing, it was common for nurses to prioritize physical care over emotional needs. However, research and experience have shown us the detrimental effects of neglecting these crucial aspects of care.

During the 19th century, notable figures such as Florence Nightingale challenged the status quo by emphasizing the importance of empathy and compassion in nursing. Nightingale's revolutionary approach to nursing focused not only on the physical wellbeing of patients but also on their emotional and psychological states. She understood that true healing occurred when patients felt seen, heard, and cared for on a holistic level.

Today, empathetic presence is firmly embedded within nursing practice. Numerous studies confirm its positive impact on patient experiences and outcomes. When nurses are present and empathetic, they form strong connections with their patients, fostering trust and understanding. This connection creates a safe space for patients to express fears, concerns, and emotions, allowing nurses to tailor care to individual needs.

When I first encountered the concept of empathetic presence, I admit that I struggled to fully understand its importance. It was easy to view it as a soft skill that came naturally to some and required effort from others. However, as I progressed in my nursing practice, I came to realise that empathetic presence is not merely a skill, but a mindset and a way of being.

Being present means fully engaging in the moment, setting aside distractions and external pressures. Only when we are truly present can we listen deeply to our patients, hear what is unspoken, and recognise their silent calls for help. Through this level of listening, we begin to understand the complex emotions and experiences our patients bring with them.

Presence alone, however, is not enough. Empathy requires us to place ourselves in our patients' positions and imagine what they may be feeling. It is the ability to understand their emotions without judgement or bias. When presence and empathy are combined, they create a powerful approach that can transform the way we care for our patients.

One of the most significant ways in which being present and empathetic enhances the care of nursing is through improved patient satisfaction. When patients feel that their emotional and psychological needs are recognised and addressed, they are more likely to feel satisfied with their overall care experience. This sense of satisfaction can lead to increased patient compliance and cooperation, ultimately contributing to improved health outcomes.

Furthermore, being present and empathetic enables nurses to better understand the unique needs of each individual patient. As we listen and observe, we gain insight into the fears, anxieties, and hopes that shape their lived experience. Equipped with this understanding, we can tailor care plans to address emotional and psychological needs, supporting holistic healing.

In my practice, I have witnessed many instances where being present and empathetic has made a meaningful difference in a patient's journey towards recovery. I recall a patient named Susan who was admitted to hospital following a severe car accident. Physically, she was healing well, but emotionally, she was struggling. She was troubled by memories of the accident and felt overwhelmed by fear and anxiety.

Initially, Peta was hesitant to open up about her emotions. It was evident that she did not want to burden others with her pain. However, I made a conscious effort to be fully present during our interactions, offering my undivided attention and demonstrating genuine empathy. Gradually, Peta began to trust me and started to share her deepest fears and concerns.

With this newfound knowledge, I was able to design a care plan that addressed Peta's emotional needs. I coordinated with the hospital's mental health team to provide her with counselling and therapy sessions. I also ensured that her room had a calming environment, incorporating elements like soothing music and aromatherapy. Over time, Peta began to regain her emotional stability, and her physical healing progressed as well.

Peta's case is just one example of how being present and empathetic can significantly enhance the car of nursing. When we make a conscious effort to be fully present with our patients, we create a safe and nurturing space for them to share their deepest fears and emotions. We validate their experiences, providing them with the support they need to navigate their healing journey.

Through empathy, we tap into the universal human experience of suffering and find common ground with our patients. We show them that they are not alone in their pain, that we are there to walk alongside them, providing solace and comfort. This shared connection creates a healing environment that extends beyond physical care, promoting the overall wellbeing of our patients.

In conclusion, being present and empathetic is more than a concept in nursing. It is a fundamental component of delivering high-quality care. By fully immersing ourselves in each moment and approaching every patient with genuine empathy, we build strong connections that encourage trust, understanding, and healing. Through empathetic presence, we enhance the care of nursing by addressing emotional and psychological needs and supporting truly holistic care.

Kindness in Action:

Kindness is an essential quality that underpins the very fabric of nursing. It flows through every interaction, every touch, and every word spoken. Kindness in action is the expression of compassion, the practice of empathy, and a powerful contributor to healing. As a nurse, I have witnessed the remarkable impact of small acts of kindness on the patient experience. In this chapter, I explore various ways nurses can demonstrate kindness and embody compassion in their practice.

1. Active listening:

One of the greatest gifts we can offer our patients is our full attention. Active listening is a simple yet meaningful act of kindness that can profoundly affect a patient's experience. It involves not only hearing their words, but also understanding their thoughts, fears, and concerns. By actively listening, we validate patients' experiences, empower them to express their needs, and create a safe space for open and honest communication.

Consider a patient who has just received a life-changing diagnosis. Their world may feel shattered as they grapple with shock, fear, and uncertainty. In this moment, active listening can provide comfort and reassurance. By sitting with them, maintaining eye contact, and listening with intent, we build trust and compassion. We give them permission to share their emotions, knowing they are heard and supported. Active listening is not about fixing problems, but about being present.

2. Providing emotional support:

As nurses, we care not only for the body but also for the emotional and spiritual wellbeing of our patients. Providing emotional support is an act of kindness that can bring immense comfort to those who are going through difficult times.

Imagine a patient who has recently lost a loved one. Their grief is overwhelming, and they feel a profound sense of emptiness and despair. In such moments, our role as nurses extends beyond administering medications and monitoring vital signs. We become conduits of solace, offering a shoulder to lean on and a hand to hold. We sit with them in their pain, providing a listening ear and a compassionate heart. By offering our presence and empathy, we help them navigate the tumultuous waters of grief and find moments of solace amidst the storm.

3. Advocating for patients:

Within a complex healthcare system, patients can often feel overwhelmed and powerless. Nurses have a vital role in advocating for their patients' rights and needs. Advocacy is a powerful act of kindness that lies at the heart of nursing practice.

Imagine a patient who is struggling to have their concerns heard by the medical team. They feel unheard and invisible, their voice drowned out by the noise of bureaucracy. In this instance, our role as advocates becomes crucial. We step up and speak up, amplifying the patient's voice and ensuring that their needs are addressed. Whether it is advocating for pain management, facilitating communication between different healthcare providers, or requesting second opinions, our advocacy acts as a protective shield that guards the interests and well-being of our patients.

4. Going the extra mile:

Nursing is often a demanding and fast-paced profession, with high patient loads and overwhelming tasks. However, going the extra mile is an act of kindness that can breathe life into the routine and elevate the patient experience. It involves stepping outside our comfort zones, pushing past the boundaries of our job descriptions, and finding innovative ways to provide exceptional care.

Imagine a patient who is feeling frightened and lonely in a hospital ward. They long for a familiar face, a comforting presence amidst the sterile walls. In this moment, going the extra mile can make a lasting impact. It may involve taking a few extra minutes to sit with the patient, engaging in meaningful conversation, or even bringing in a small memento from home to create a sense of familiarity. Going the extra mile is about recognizing the humanity in every patient and acknowledging that their needs extend beyond mere medical interventions.

Small gestures of kindness:

Often, it is the smallest gestures that have the greatest impact. A warm blanket, a cup of tea, or a genuine smile can bring comfort and reassurance. These acts can shift a patient's experience from one of detachment to one of warmth and connection.

Consider a patient confined to bed for days, feeling disconnected from the outside world. A simple gesture, such as arranging flowers, offering a book, or holding their hand during a painful procedure, can restore a sense of dignity and hope. These moments remind patients that they are seen, valued, and cared for.

The CAR of Nursing

Kindness in action is the essence of nursing. It is the guiding force behind every compassionate nurse. Through active listening, emotional support, patient advocacy, going the extra mile, and offering small acts of kindness, we embody the true spirit of care. We become the CAR of nursing: compassionate, attentive, and responsive to the needs of those entrusted to us. Through kindness, we create healing environments, empower our patients, and leave a lasting impact on their lives.

Building Trust and Rapport:

Trust and rapport are the cornerstones of effective nursing practice. As a clinical nurse with many years of nursing, my primary goal is to establish and maintain a compassionate relationship with my patients, allowing them to feel safe and valued during their time of need. In this chapter, I will delve into the significance of trust and rapport within nursing, exploring the ways in which these components lay the foundation for holistic care.

Trust is the bedrock upon which all relationships are built. In the realm of nursing, it is the essence that allows patients to feel secure in the presence of their healthcare providers. Establishing trust with patients goes beyond the clinical skills and knowledge we possess. It requires active listening, empathy, and genuine compassion. Through myriad personal experiences, I have come to realize that trust must be earned and nurtured. Patients often arrive at the hospital feeling vulnerable, scared, and unsure about what lies ahead. It is through our actions and words that we can instill a sense of trust, letting patients know that they are in capable, caring hands.

Rapport, on the other hand, refers to the interpersonal connection that develops between nurses and patients. Through rapport, mutual understanding is established, supporting open communication and collaboration. Building rapport is an ongoing process that requires active participation from both nurse and patient. By listening attentively, showing empathy, and respecting each patient's individuality, nurses can develop strong therapeutic relationships. Rapport enhances patient comfort and creates an environment in which patients feel confident sharing their concerns, fears, and personal experiences.

The importance of trust and rapport in nursing cannot be underestimated. These elements not only influence the overall patient experience but also affect the success of treatments and interventions. Research has shown that patients who trust their healthcare providers are more likely to follow medical advice and treatment plans, leading to improved health outcomes. In addition, the presence of strong rapport has been shown to reduce patient anxiety and increase satisfaction. Trust and rapport are therefore not abstract concepts, but essential components of effective nursing care.

To build trust and rapport, one must be mindful of their words, actions, and non-verbal cues. Every interaction with a patient has the potential to make a lasting impression. As a nurse, I have learned that the power of a simple smile, a gentle touch, or a reassuring word can go a long way in establishing a connection with patients. By creating a comfortable and welcoming environment, we can foster an atmosphere where patients can openly express their concerns and feel heard. Through active listening, we validate their feelings, allowing them to know that they are being taken seriously.

One effective approach to building trust and rapport is to remain authentic and sincere in all interactions. Patients are often perceptive and can sense when behaviour lacks genuineness. By demonstrating empathy and honesty, we create a safe space that allows patients to lower their defences and place trust in our care. It is important to remember that trust is not built in a single moment. It is an ongoing process that requires consistency, reliability, and commitment. Nurses must continually demonstrate trustworthiness by following through on promises and maintaining open communication.

Furthermore, it is important to recognize that building trust and rapport is not a one-size-fits-all approach. Each patient brings their unique background, experiences, and beliefs to the healthcare encounter. As nurses, it is our responsibility to respect and honour these differences, cherishing the diversity that exists within our patient population. By taking the time to understand and acknowledge the individuality of each patient, we can tailor our approach to ensure a personalized and compassionate experience.

In conclusion, trust and rapport serve as the foundation for compassionate relationships in nursing. By building trust, we create an environment where patients can feel safe and valued, promoting their engagement in their own care. Rapport, on the other hand, facilitates open communication and collaboration, allowing for holistic and patient-cantered care. As nurses, we must recognize the importance of these components and continuously strive to cultivate trust and rapport with every patient we encounter. By doing so, we will not only enhance the patient experience but also contribute to better health outcomes and the overall well-being of those in our care.

Compassion Fatigue:

As a nurse, I have witnessed firsthand the significant challenges and demands associated with caring for patients. We dedicate ourselves to supporting others, advocating for them, and providing comfort during times of illness and vulnerability. However, in focusing so heavily on the needs of others, we can often neglect our own wellbeing, leading to a condition known as compassion fatigue.

Compassion fatigue refers to the emotional and physical exhaustion experienced by healthcare providers as a result of prolonged exposure to patient suffering and traumatic situations. It is not a sign of weakness or lack of competence, but rather a natural response to the demanding nature of the profession. Continuous exposure to pain, distress, and trauma can affect our mental, emotional, and physical health, and may ultimately result in burnout if not addressed.

To manage and prevent compassion fatigue, it is essential for nurses to recognise its signs and develop effective coping strategies. Awareness of emotional limits and the impact of our work on personal wellbeing is critical. This requires a shift in perspective, recognising that prioritising self-care and seeking support is both appropriate and necessary. We must remember that effective care for others begins with caring for ourselves.

Recognising the Signs and Symptoms of Compassion Fatigue:

Compassion fatigue can manifest in various ways, and recognizing the signs and symptoms is the first step towards prevention and management. Some common signs include feelings of emotional exhaustion, increased cynicism or detachment from patients, decreased job satisfaction, difficulty sleeping, irritability, and even physical symptoms like headaches or stomach-aches. By being aware of these indicators, we can intervene early and prevent compassion fatigue from progressing.

Prevention Strategies for Compassion Fatigue:

Prevention is always preferable to treatment, and this is particularly true for compassion fatigue. Implementing proactive strategies can help build resilience and reduce risk. The following strategies have proven beneficial in my experience:

1. **Self-care:** Make self-care a priority in daily life. This may include activities that promote relaxation and enjoyment, such as exercise, reading, spending time with loved ones, or engaging in hobbies. Taking regular breaks and scheduled leave is also essential for recovery and renewal.

2. **Establish boundaries:** Set clear boundaries in both professional and personal contexts. It is acceptable to decline additional responsibilities when feeling overwhelmed. Establishing realistic expectations and learning to delegate tasks can significantly reduce stress.

3. **Seek support:** Develop a strong support network of colleagues, friends, coaches, or mentors who understand the demands of nursing. Sharing experiences and coping strategies with others can provide valuable emotional support.

4. **Practise mindfulness:** Incorporate mindfulness practices into daily routines. This may include meditation, breathing exercises, or moments of reflection and gratitude. Mindfulness can help reduce stress and improve emotional resilience.

Management Strategies for Compassion Fatigue:

Despite strong preventative measures, there may still be times when compassion fatigue occurs. In such cases, effective management strategies are essential:

1. **Self-reflection:** Take time to reflect on emotions and experiences related to work. Journalling can help process feelings and identify stress triggers, supporting greater self-awareness and recovery.

2. **Professional support:** Seek professional assistance through counselling or therapy. Speaking with a trained professional provides a safe space to explore emotions, develop coping strategies, seek feedback from line managers, and gain fresh perspectives.

3. **Self-compassion:** Treat yourself with the same kindness and understanding offered to patients. Acknowledge the challenges of the role and accept that feeling overwhelmed at times is normal. Practising self-compassion supports emotional recovery and wellbeing.

4. **Work-life balance:** Review the balance between professional responsibilities and personal life. Consider adjustments that may reduce stress and allow more time for self-care. This may include changes to work schedules, seeking workplace support, or exploring professional development opportunities to improve job satisfaction.

In conclusion, addressing compassion fatigue is of utmost importance in maintaining the well-being of nurses. By recognizing the signs and symptoms, implementing prevention strategies, and practicing effective management techniques, we can combat compassion fatigue and continue to provide the quality care our patients deserve. Remember, compassion starts with ourselves, and by taking care of our own well-being, we can be more compassionate caregivers.

Chapter 9:
The Engine of Knowledge

Evidence-based Practice

Incorporating evidence-based practice into our daily routine as nurses means consistently striving to base our interventions and treatments on the most current and reliable research. This approach not only improves patient outcomes but also enhances patient safety and supports the delivery of high-quality care. It ensures that the care we provide is grounded in scientific evidence rather than outdated or unsupported practices.

One of the key advantages of evidence-based practice is its ability to bridge the gap between research and clinical practice. Through this approach, research findings can be effectively translated into everyday nursing care. This ensures that nursing interventions are not based solely on opinion or tradition, but on evidence that has been rigorously evaluated and validated.

To adopt evidence-based practice, I have learned the importance of critically appraising research studies and assessing their relevance to my clinical setting. This skill allows me to evaluate the quality and credibility of research articles, ensuring that clinical decisions are informed by dependable evidence. By analysing research strengths and limitations, I can determine which interventions are most appropriate for my patients.

Implementing evidence-based practice in nursing requires a commitment to continuous learning and improvement. As nurses, we are dedicated to staying informed about emerging research and incorporating new evidence into our practice. This commitment ensures that care delivery evolves alongside advances in healthcare. It also encourages a culture of lifelong learning within the profession, where nurses are motivated to question existing practices and seek better ways to improve patient care.

The CAR of Nursing

By embracing evidence-based practice, we can confidently provide care that is supported by scientific evidence. This approach empowers us to justify our decisions and interventions to both our patients and my colleagues. It also allows us to advocate for the adoption of evidence-based practice within the healthcare setting, as we can confidently assert that the interventions we provide are grounded in reliable research and are in the best interest of our patients.

Evidence-based practice is not without its challenges. As a nurse, I have encountered resistance from colleagues who may be sceptical about the value of evidence-based practice or find it difficult to incorporate into their own practices. However, I firmly believe that evidence-based practice is the cornerstone of delivering quality care and improving patient outcomes. Therefore, I am dedicated to promoting its importance and supporting my colleagues in the adoption of evidence-based practice.

As the field of nursing continues to evolve, evidence-based practice will remain an essential component of delivering the highest standard of care. The ever-expanding body of research and evidence necessitates that nurses remain diligent in their commitment to evidence-based practice. By continuously seeking out the most current and reliable evidence, critically appraising research studies, and applying the findings to their practice, nurses can ensure that they are delivering care that is consistent with the latest advancements in healthcare.

In conclusion, evidence-based practice is more than just a buzzword in the nursing profession. It is a fundamental approach to delivering quality care that is supported by scientific evidence. By incorporating evidence-based practice into our daily routine as nurses, we can ensure that our interventions and treatments are based on the most up-to-date and reliable research. This approach improves patient outcomes, enhances patient safety, and promotes the delivery of high-quality care. Furthermore, evidence-based practice bridges the gap between research and clinical practice, ensuring that nursing interventions are grounded in scientific evidence. It encourages nurses to critically appraise research studies and apply the findings to their practice, fostering a culture of continuous learning and improvement within the nursing profession. As a nurse, I am committed to embracing evidence-based practice and advocating for its importance in delivering the best possible care to my patients.

Continuing Education

Throughout history, nursing has undergone significant advancement and transformation. In its early years, nursing was often viewed as a vocation, with limited emphasis on formal education or professional development. Training occurred largely on the job, guided by experience and senior healthcare professionals. As healthcare systems became more complex and specialised, the need for structured education and ongoing learning became increasingly clear.

The concept of continuing education for nurses began to gain recognition in the mid-20th century. It was during this time that nursing education underwent significant changes, transitioning from hospital-based training programs to formal academic programs offered by educational institutions. This shift marked the recognition of nursing as a profession, requiring a solid foundation of knowledge and skills.

As the profession evolved, lifelong learning and professional development became central to nursing practice. Nurses recognised that maintaining high standards of care required continual updates to knowledge and skills in line with best practice and evidence-based guidelines. The rapid growth of medical knowledge reinforced the need for ongoing education to remain current and competent.

One of the key advantages of lifelong learning and professional development is the opportunity it provides for nurses to enhance their competence and expertise. Through continuing education, nurses can deepen their understanding of complex medical conditions, develop specialized skills, and refine their clinical judgment. This not only benefits the nurse personally but also has a direct positive impact on patient outcomes.

The CAR of Nursing

Continuing education also serves as a vehicle for professional growth and career advancement. With new knowledge and skills acquired through ongoing learning, nurses can pursue specialized roles, such as critical care nursing or advanced practice nursing. These advanced roles come with increased responsibilities and require a higher level of expertise. Continuing education empowers nurses to take on these roles with confidence, knowing that they are equipped with the latest knowledge and skills necessary to excel.

Another key aspect of lifelong learning is its role in promoting evidence-based practice. In healthcare, evidence-based practice involves combining research evidence, clinical expertise, and patient preferences. By engaging in continuing education, nurses remain informed about current research and can integrate evidence-based approaches into their care. This leads to improved patient outcomes and enhances the overall quality of healthcare delivery.

Continuing education also plays a crucial role in maintaining professional standards and complying with regulatory requirements. In many countries, nursing regulatory bodies require nurses to complete a certain number of continuing education hours within a specific time frame to renew their licenses. This serves as a mechanism to ensure that nurses remain competent in their practice and are up to date with the evolving standards of care. By engaging in lifelong learning and professional development, nurses demonstrate their commitment to maintaining high professional standards and providing safe and effective care.

Moreover, continuing education facilitates interdisciplinary collaboration and knowledge sharing. In today's healthcare environment, teamwork and collaboration are essential for providing comprehensive patient care. Through continuing education activities, nurses can interact with healthcare professionals from different disciplines and learn from their perspectives. For example, in the rehabilitation unit, Logan hospital where I work, we allocated 30 minutes each day for in-service for nursing staff. This exchange of knowledge and experiences fosters a culture of collaboration and promotes a holistic approach to patient care.

Continuing education can take many forms, including academic study, workshops, conferences, seminars, webinars, and online learning. The choice of learning activities depends on individual preferences, availability, and professional goals. It is essential for nurses to actively seek learning opportunities and invest in their ongoing development.

In conclusion, lifelong learning and professional development are essential for nurses to succeed in their careers and deliver high-quality care. Through continuing education, nurses enhance competence, pursue specialised roles, support evidence-based practice, meet regulatory requirements, and collaborate effectively with multidisciplinary teams. As a nurse, I am committed to continuous learning and staying informed about current knowledge and best practice. By doing so, I can continue to make a meaningful contribution to patient care and support the advancement of the nursing profession.

Critical Thinking Skills:

First and foremost, critical thinking skills enable us to navigate the complex world of clinical decision-making. Nurses are frequently faced with challenging situations that require careful attention and thoughtful analysis. With strong critical thinking skills, we can assess these situations by systematically gathering relevant information and data. This process allows us to make informed decisions about patient care. As a result, we are able to deliver safe and effective nursing interventions, supporting the health and wellbeing of those entrusted to our care.

Furthermore, critical thinking skills empower us to solve problems efficiently and effectively. Our role as nurses is not limited to mere caretakers; we are problem solvers. A strong foundation in critical thinking enables us to identify the needs of our patients, no matter how subtle, and take proactive measures to address them. We are skilled at assessing potential complications and formulating care plans that are tailored to each individual patient's unique circumstances. With this skillset, we can avert potential complications before they arise, providing the highest level of care possible.

The CAR of Nursing

In addition to problem-solving, critical thinking skills strengthen our role as patient advocates. Nurses are often the voice for individuals who may struggle to speak for themselves. Through careful evaluation of clinical information and available evidence, we ensure that patients receive the most appropriate and effective care. By involving patients in decision-making, we empower them to take an active role in their own health. This advocacy is a fundamental aspect of nursing and highlights the importance of critical thinking in clinical practice.

Effective communication is yet another area in which critical thinking skills play a significant role. As nurses, we are tasked with conveying complex medical concepts to patients, their families, and other healthcare professionals. It is through critical analysis and interpretation of information that we can distil these concepts into clear and understandable language. We must be able to communicate with empathy, ensuring that our patients feel heard and understood. By mastering the art of effective communication, we foster an environment of trust and collaboration, enhancing the quality of care we provide.

Beyond the immediate impact on patient care, critical thinking skills also encourage us as nurses to engage in continuous learning and professional development. Our profession is dynamic and ever-changing, and to remain at the cutting edge, we must constantly seek out new knowledge and advancements. Critical thinking skills enable us to critically evaluate new research findings, evidence-based practices, and technological innovations. We become the conduits of progress, continuously striving to enhance our knowledge and skills to better serve our patients and the nursing profession.

In conclusion, critical thinking skills form the foundation of nursing practice. They underpin our ability to deliver high-quality, evidence-based care while maintaining patient safety. These skills enable us to navigate the complex challenges we face, propelling us forward as problem solvers and advocates for those in our care. Effective communication and continuous learning are essential components of our practice, facilitated by our capacity for critical analysis and reflection. As nurses, we must recognize the indispensable role that critical thinking skills play in our profession, embracing their power and potential. By doing so, we will continue to elevate the practice of nursing, advancing healthcare and welfare for all.

Chapter 10:
The Steering Wheel of Leadership

Transformational Leadership:

To truly understand the concept of transformational leadership, it is essential to compare it with other leadership styles. Traditional leadership approaches, such as autocratic or transactional leadership, typically prioritise task completion and adhere to a hierarchical structure. In these models, leaders rely on rewards and punishments to motivate their followers. While these styles may be effective in certain situations, they often fall short in fostering employee engagement and personal growth.

In contrast, transformational leadership takes a holistic approach, placing a strong emphasis on building relationships, fostering trust, and empowering individuals. Transformational leaders strive to inspire and motivate their followers by creating a compelling vision, setting clear goals, and providing the necessary support and guidance for their teams. They create a sense of purpose and belonging, enabling individuals to surpass their own expectations and achieve exceptional outcomes.

The impact of transformational leadership on nursing practice is profound. It has the potential to enhance job satisfaction and engagement among nurses, resulting in increased productivity and improved patient outcomes. When nurses feel supported and valued, it elevates their level of commitment and encourages them to go the extra mile for their patients. By recognising and rewarding excellence, transformational leaders create a culture of high performance, where nurses are more likely to take initiative and innovate in their practice.

Moreover, the essence of transformational leadership lies in the ability to form strong and trusting relationships. When leaders invest time and effort in getting to know their team members on a personal level, it fosters a sense of camaraderie and collaboration. This, in turn, leads to effective communication and coordination among healthcare professionals, ultimately enhancing patient care. A united front of nurses, motivated by their transformational leader, can create a harmonious environment where everyone's skills and expertise are utilised for the benefit of patients.

Transformational leaders also understand the importance of nurturing their staff's professional development and growth. By providing opportunities for education and skill enhancement, leaders empower their team members to continually improve their practice. This investment in their development not only benefits the individual nurse but also contributes to the overall advancement of the nursing profession. Creating a culture of continuous learning and innovation ensures that the nursing workforce remains up to date with the latest evidence-based practices and plays a pivotal role in shaping the future of healthcare.

One of the remarkable aspects of transformational leadership is its ability to instil a sense of ownership and accountability among nurses. When individuals are inspired by their leader's vision and have a clear understanding of their role in achieving it, they become more invested in their work. This ownership leads to increased job satisfaction and a willingness to take responsibility for their actions. Nurses under the guidance of a transformational leader are more likely to exhibit a strong work ethic, integrity, and a commitment to delivering exceptional patient care.

It is important to note that transformational leadership is not limited to those in formal leadership positions. It is a mindset that can be adopted by anyone, regardless of their title or rank. In fact, transformational leadership can be particularly impactful at the bedside, where nurses are directly involved in patient care. By embracing the principles of transformational leadership, nurses can create a positive and supportive environment for their colleagues, fostering collaboration and empowering each other to provide the best possible care.

In conclusion, transformational leadership has the potential to revolutionise the field of nursing. Its ability to inspire and motivate individuals to reach their full potential has a profound impact on nursing practice. By fostering a sense of purpose, building trust, and investing in the professional development of their teams, transformational leaders create a culture of excellence and innovation. The ripple effects of transformational leadership extend beyond the workplace, benefiting both nurses and patients alike. It is through this style of leadership that we can truly elevate the art and science of nursing and pave the way for a brighter future in healthcare.

Effective Communication in Leadership:

To truly understand the role of effective communication in leadership, it is vital to explore its historical timeline. Communication has always been an integral part of human civilisation, serving as a means of conveying thoughts, ideas, and emotions. In ancient times, leaders relied heavily on verbal communication, with words being of utmost importance. Oral traditions passed down stories, knowledge, and wisdom from one generation to the next. This oral transmission allowed leaders to inspire their followers, rallying them around a common cause.

With the advent of writing systems, leadership communication expanded its boundaries. The written word became a powerful tool for conveying information, ensuring its accuracy and longevity. Ancient leaders etched their decrees, laws, and philosophies onto stone tablets, papyrus scrolls, and later, paper. These written communications were disseminated among the populace, shaping individual and collective beliefs.

However, it was not until the emergence of the printing press that leadership communication gained unprecedented reach and influence. The ability to mass produce written materials in the fifteenth century revolutionised communication, as stories, ideas, and scientific discoveries could now be shared with a wider audience. This advancement allowed leaders to disseminate their messages more efficiently, leading to societal transformations and the acceleration of knowledge.

Fast forward to the twenty-first century, and we find ourselves in the midst of a digital revolution that has forever changed the landscape of leadership communication. With the advent of the internet, leaders now have a multitude of channels at their disposal to connect with their team members and stakeholders. Email, instant messaging, video conferencing, social media platforms, and other communication tools have revolutionised the way leaders interact and share information.

In nursing leadership, effective communication is paramount. Building trust with the nursing team is foundational for a leader's success. Trust is earned through open and transparent communication, where leaders convey information honestly, without hidden agendas or ulterior motives. By establishing trust through effective communication, leaders inspire confidence among their team members, foster collaboration, and create a supportive environment conducive to growth and achievement.

Clear direction is another crucial aspect of effective leadership communication. Nurses look to their leaders for guidance and direction in navigating the complex healthcare landscape. Effective leaders communicate clear goals and expectations, ensuring that every team member understands their role and responsibilities. This clarity of direction aligns everyone towards a common objective, promoting unity and synergy within the nursing team.

Collaboration and teamwork are essential in nursing, as patient care often requires a multidisciplinary approach. Effective communication fosters an environment where open dialogue, active listening, and the sharing of ideas are encouraged. Leaders with strong communication skills can facilitate productive discussions where each team member's unique perspective is valued. This collaborative approach to problem-solving and decision-making enhances patient care outcomes and promotes a culture of innovation.

Conflict resolution is another critical aspect of effective leadership communication. In nursing, conflicts may arise due to differences in opinions, work styles, or competing priorities. Leaders who possess effective communication skills can address conflicts in a timely and constructive manner. By facilitating open and honest discussions, leaders can identify the underlying issues, explore potential solutions, and mediate disputes. This proactive approach to conflict resolution prevents disagreements from escalating, preserves team dynamics, and ensures a harmonious working environment.

Furthermore, effective communication plays a pivotal role in motivating and engaging nursing personnel. Nurses work in a demanding and high-stress environment, where burnout and disengagement can occur. Leaders who communicate effectively regularly provide feedback, recognising individual achievements and offering support when needed. By acknowledging the contributions of team members and promoting a positive work environment, leaders foster motivation and engagement among the nursing staff.

Building and Motivating Teams:

To truly understand the significance of building and motivating teams, it is essential to first grasp the definition of a team in the nursing context. A nursing team comprises individuals from various backgrounds, each with unique skill sets and expertise, working together towards a common goal: optimal patient outcomes. This collaboration is built on trust, respect, and effective communication, and it is the responsibility of nurse leaders to nurture and develop these qualities within their teams.

One of the fundamental strategies for building an effective nursing team is to clearly define the team's purpose and goals. When team members are aware of the bigger picture and understand how their individual roles contribute to the overall objectives, they are more likely to be motivated and engaged in their work. As a nurse leader, it is crucial to communicate this purpose effectively and consistently, ensuring that every team member feels valued and understands the impact they have on patient care.

In addition to establishing a sense of purpose, creating a supportive and inclusive environment is vital for building and motivating nursing teams. Recognising and acknowledging the unique contributions of each team member fosters a sense of belonging and boosts morale. Regular team meetings and huddles provide an opportunity for open and honest communication, allowing team members to voice their concerns, share ideas, and provide feedback. This open dialogue not only strengthens relationships between team members but also allows for continuous improvement and growth.

Another effective strategy for motivating nursing teams is through the implementation of a reward and recognition program. Celebrating individual and team accomplishments, no matter how small, can have a profound impact on employee satisfaction and morale. Recognising the efforts and achievements of team members not only reinforces positive behaviour but also encourages others to strive for excellence. Nurse leaders should understand the preferences and interests of their team members, tailoring rewards and recognition to align with their individual motivations.

Moreover, building effective nursing teams requires investment in the professional development of team members. Providing opportunities for continuous learning and growth not only enhances the skills and knowledge of individual nurses but also improves their confidence and job satisfaction. Nurse leaders can support professional development by offering educational resources, sponsoring conferences and workshops, and facilitating mentorship programs. By investing in the growth of their team members, nurse leaders not only motivate their teams but also ensure the delivery of high-quality patient care.

Furthermore, building and motivating effective nursing teams also involves fostering a culture of collaboration and teamwork. Encouraging interdisciplinary collaboration and creating opportunities for cross-functional projects and initiatives allows team members to gain a broader perspective of patient care. This collaboration not only improves patient outcomes but also enhances the professional growth of individual team members. Nurse leaders should promote a culture of shared decision-making, mutual respect, and active engagement, facilitating effective teamwork and enabling optimal patient care delivery.

Lastly, effective leadership plays a pivotal role in building and motivating nursing teams. A nurse leader's influence extends far beyond their own actions; they must serve as role models for excellence, integrity, and professionalism. Nurse leaders must possess strong communication and interpersonal skills, building relationships based on trust and respect. By understanding the strengths and weaknesses of their team members, nurse leaders can assign tasks and responsibilities accordingly, maximising individual contributions and fostering a sense of empowerment.

In conclusion, building and motivating effective nursing teams is a multifaceted process that requires intentional effort and investment from nurse leaders. By clearly defining the team's purpose and goals, creating a supportive and inclusive environment, implementing reward and recognition programs, investing in professional development, fostering a culture of collaboration, and demonstrating effective leadership, nurse leaders can cultivate empowered and motivated nursing teams. Through these strategies, nurse leaders can improve patient outcomes, enhance job satisfaction, and create a positive and productive work environment in the healthcare setting.

Conflict Resolution:

Conflict in the nursing profession is not a novel concept. Throughout history, nurses have faced challenges and conflicts within their professional relationships. By examining the historical timeline of conflict resolution in nursing, we can gain insight into how professionals have worked to address and overcome these issues.

In the early years of nursing, conflict was often suppressed and ignored. Nurses were expected to conform to a strict hierarchy, and any disagreements were seen as a sign of incompetence or insubordination. This approach to conflict stifled creativity and hindered the growth of the profession.

During the mid-twentieth century, the nursing profession underwent significant changes. With the rise of nursing organisations and unions, nurses began to assert their rights and voice their concerns. This newfound assertiveness led to an increase in conflicts within the profession. Nurses demanded better working conditions, fair compensation, and opportunities for professional growth.

As the profession evolved, so did the strategies for conflict resolution. The advent of nursing research and evidence-based practice provided a foundation for resolving conflicts through a systematic approach. Nurses began to utilise communication techniques and problem-solving models to address conflicts effectively.

In today's healthcare environment, nurses are expected to work collaboratively as part of a multidisciplinary team. This dynamic often leads to conflicts arising from differing perspectives, priorities, and values. To address these conflicts, it is crucial for nurses to first acknowledge and understand the underlying issues.

One effective strategy for conflict resolution is open and honest communication. By openly discussing the conflict and actively listening to each party's concerns, nurses can gain a deeper understanding of the issue at hand. This transparency can help bridge the gap between conflicting parties and foster a sense of mutual respect and understanding.

Another essential aspect of conflict resolution is the ability to identify and address the emotions involved. Conflicts can elicit strong emotions such as frustration, anger, and resentment. It is important for nurses to recognise these emotions and find healthy ways to manage them. This may involve seeking support from supervisors or colleagues, practising self-care techniques, or utilising stress-reducing strategies.

Collaboration and compromise are at the heart of effective conflict resolution. Nurses must be willing to find common ground and work together to reach a mutually beneficial solution. This may require brainstorming ideas, exploring alternative perspectives, and finding creative ways to meet everyone's needs.

In some cases, conflicts within the nursing profession may be deeply rooted in systemic issues. Nurses may find themselves facing conflicts stemming from issues such as lack of resources, understaffing, or policy constraints. In these situations, it is important for nurses to advocate for change and work towards addressing the underlying issues. This may involve engaging in collective bargaining, participating in quality improvement initiatives, or advocating for policy changes at the organisational or legislative level.

Conflict resolution in nursing is not a one-size-fits-all approach. Each conflict is unique, and the strategies employed may vary depending on the individuals involved and the nature of the conflict. However, by fostering open communication, addressing emotions, and promoting collaboration, nurses can work towards resolving conflicts in a constructive and productive manner.

As nurses, we have a responsibility to create a positive and supportive work environment. By mastering the art of conflict resolution, we can foster healthy relationships, enhance patient care, and contribute to the overall success of the profession. Conflict will always be a part of the nursing profession, as we are all human, but with the right skills and strategies, we can transform these conflicts into opportunities for growth and improvement.

Inspiring Change and Innovation:

One of the most important reasons to highlight the importance of inspiring change and fostering innovation in nursing practice is the ever-changing nature of healthcare itself. Medical knowledge is constantly expanding, and new technologies are being developed at a rapid pace. As nurses, it is our responsibility to stay at the forefront of these advancements and incorporate them into our practice. By doing so, we can ensure that we are providing the highest quality care to our patients.

In addition to keeping up with advancements in medical knowledge and technology, inspiring change and fostering innovation in nursing practice can also lead to improved patient outcomes. By embracing new approaches and techniques, we can find more effective ways to treat and care for our patients. For example, by implementing evidence-based practice, we can ensure that our interventions are based on the best available evidence and tailored to each individual patient's needs. This can result in faster recoveries, reduced complications, and overall better patient satisfaction.

Furthermore, inspiring change and fostering innovation in nursing practice can also lead to increased efficiency and cost savings in healthcare. This is particularly important in today's healthcare landscape, where resources are often limited. By identifying areas for improvement and implementing innovative solutions, we can streamline processes, reduce waste, and ultimately save both time and money. For example, by introducing new technologies or approaches to documentation, we can simplify workflows and improve communication between healthcare providers, leading to more efficient and effective patient care.

Another crucial aspect of inspiring change and fostering innovation in nursing practice is the impact it can have on nursing as a profession. Nursing is a dynamic field that requires constant adaptation and growth. By inspiring change and fostering innovation, we can attract and retain talented individuals who are eager to contribute to the advancement of nursing practice. This can result in a more diverse and skilled workforce, capable of meeting the complex needs of today's patients.

Inspiring change and fostering innovation in nursing practice can also help to address some of the key challenges and issues facing healthcare today. For example, the nursing shortage is a pressing concern in many parts of the world. By embracing innovative staffing models and exploring new ways to attract and retain nurses, we can help to alleviate the burden on the healthcare system and ensure that patients receive the care they deserve.

Moreover, inspiring change and fostering innovation in nursing practice can also help to address disparities in healthcare and promote health equity. By identifying and addressing the underlying factors contributing to these disparities, such as bias and discrimination, we can work towards creating a more just and equitable healthcare system. This requires a willingness to challenge the status quo and actively advocate for change.

In conclusion, inspiring change and fostering innovation in nursing practice is of paramount importance in today's healthcare landscape.

The CAR of Nursing

By embracing new knowledge and technologies, improving patient outcomes, increasing efficiency, advancing the nursing profession, and addressing key challenges, we can ensure that we are providing the best possible care to our patients. It is up to every one of us as nurses to drive this change and be the agents of innovation that our profession needs. Together, we can make a lasting impact on healthcare and create a brighter future for nursing.

Chapter 11:
The Seat of Advocacy:

Patient Rights and Autonomy:

Patient rights are based on the principle that individuals have the right to be informed, involved, and respected in their healthcare decisions. These rights are crucial for establishing a therapeutic relationship between the nurse and the patient, as well as for ensuring the provision of patient-centred care. When patients are aware of their rights, they are more likely to actively participate in their own care, ask questions, voice concerns, and make informed decisions. This not only improves patient satisfaction but also contributes to better health outcomes.

One of the key components of patient rights is the right to informed consent. Informed consent is a process by which healthcare professionals inform patients about the risks, benefits, and alternatives of a proposed treatment or procedure, and obtain their voluntary agreement to proceed. It is not merely a form to be signed, but a conversation that empowers the patient to make decisions based on their personal values and preferences. As a nurse, I have a responsibility to ensure that patients fully understand the information provided, including any potential risks or side effects, so that they can make truly autonomous decisions.

Promoting patient autonomy also involves respecting their right to refuse or discontinue treatment. While it can be challenging to accept a patient's decision when it may conflict with medical advice or perceived best interests, it is crucial to remember that autonomy is a fundamental human right. As nurses, we must respect and support patients in making decisions about their own bodies, even when those decisions may not align with our personal beliefs or medical opinions. This requires active listening, empathy, and providing non-judgemental support to patients as they navigate their healthcare journey.

Another aspect of patient rights and autonomy is ensuring privacy and confidentiality. Patients have the right to expect that their personal health information will be kept private and protected from unauthorised access. This not only protects their dignity and autonomy but also maintains trust between the patient and healthcare providers. As nurses, we are responsible for safeguarding patient information and only sharing it on a need-to-know basis. We must also ensure that patients are aware of their rights regarding the privacy and confidentiality of their health information and provide them with the necessary education and resources to exercise those rights.

In addition to these fundamental patient rights, healthcare organisations and professionals must also be mindful of cultural and individual diversity. Patients come from a wide range of backgrounds and may have unique cultural, religious, or personal beliefs that influence their healthcare decisions. It is important for nurses to be culturally sensitive and respectful, ensuring that patients' cultural and personal values are considered when planning and delivering care. This may involve involving interpreters, adapting care plans to respect religious beliefs or dietary preferences, or engaging in open conversations about patients' cultural practices and preferences.

Research has consistently demonstrated the positive impact of upholding patient rights and promoting autonomy in nursing. Studies have shown that patients who feel respected, involved, and informed about their care experience better overall health outcomes, are more satisfied with their healthcare experience, and are more likely to adhere to treatment plans. Additionally, promoting patient autonomy has been associated with increased patient engagement, improved patient-provider communication, and reduced healthcare disparities.

Unfortunately, without specific research papers or studies to refer to, it is not possible to provide a list of interesting points related to patient rights and autonomy in nursing. However, I can draw on my experiences and observations to highlight the significance of these principles.

The CAR of Nursing

One particularly memorable case comes to mind, where the importance of patient rights and autonomy was evident. I was caring for a patient who was diagnosed with a terminal illness. Despite the prognosis, the patient expressed a desire to explore alternative treatments and therapies. Initially, the medical team was sceptical of these alternatives and believed that the traditional treatment plan was the only viable option. However, through open and honest conversations, the patient was able to assert their autonomy and discuss their preferences, values, and goals. The patient's rights were respected, and the medical team, including myself, supported the patient in exploring complementary therapies alongside the conventional treatment plan.

This experience taught me that patient autonomy is not just about making choices, but about empowering patients to take an active role in their own care. By fostering an environment that values patient rights and autonomy, we can promote collaboration, shared decision-making, and ultimately, better health outcomes.

In conclusion, upholding patient rights and promoting autonomy is essential for effective nursing practice. Patient rights encompass principles such as informed consent, the right to refuse or discontinue treatment, and privacy and confidentiality. These rights are rooted in the fundamental idea that individuals have the right to make decisions about their own health and wellbeing. As nurses, it is our duty to respect and support patients in exercising their autonomy, regardless of our personal beliefs or medical opinions. By upholding patient rights and promoting autonomy, we can establish a therapeutic relationship, provide patient-centred care, and ultimately improve health outcomes.

Ethical Dilemmas and Decision-making:

One such dilemma that still haunts me to this day unfolded during my early years as a nurse. I was caring for a patient who had been diagnosed with terminal cancer. The prognosis was grim, and the patient's family was understandably devastated. The patient's adult children, who had power of attorney, were faced with the agonising decision of whether to continue aggressive treatment or to transition their loved one to palliative care. As healthcare professionals, we offered our expertise and guidance, but ultimately, it was their decision to make.

The ethical dilemma arose when the patient's children were divided on what course of action to take. One insisted on continuing aggressive treatment, hoping for a miraculous recovery, while the other believed that palliative care was the most compassionate option for their parent. As their nurse, I found myself caught in the middle, torn between the duty to respect the patient's autonomy and the desire to provide the best possible care.

I turned to various ethical decision-making strategies to help guide me through this challenging situation. The Four Principles Approach, which emphasises autonomy, beneficence, non-maleficence, and justice, provided a framework for evaluating the conflicting values at play. I considered the patient's right to self-determination, the potential benefits and harms of each treatment option, and the fair distribution of resources. However, this framework did not alleviate the emotional turmoil I experienced as I grappled with the weight of the decision.

To gain further clarity, I sought guidance from my colleagues and supervisor. We engaged in team discussions, exploring different perspectives and sharing our own personal experiences. These conversations helped to highlight the complexity of the situation and the various ethical considerations involved. It was during these discussions that I realised the importance of approaching ethical dilemmas as a collective effort, rather than trying to bear the burden alone.

Additionally, the ICN (International Council of Nurses) Code of Ethics served as a valuable resource in guiding my decision-making process. The code emphasises the nurse's responsibility to advocate for the patient, promote their wellbeing, and maintain their trust. It reminded me that my primary duty was to provide compassionate care and support to the patient and their family, regardless of the decision that was ultimately made.

In the end, the patient's children chose to transition their loved one to palliative care. It was a difficult decision, but one that was made with careful consideration and in accordance with the patient's wishes. As their nurse, I respected their autonomy and did everything in my power to ensure a smooth transition to palliative care. I provided emotional support to the family, communicated their concerns and preferences to the healthcare team, and facilitated open and honest conversations about end-of-life care.

This experience taught me the importance of self-reflection and ongoing professional development in the realm of ethical decision-making. It reinforced the need for nurses to be equipped with the knowledge, skills, and ethical frameworks necessary to navigate the complex moral landscape of healthcare. As I continued to grow in my career, I sought out opportunities for further education and training in ethics.

Through workshops, conferences, and online courses, I deepened my understanding of ethical principles and learned about new strategies for ethical decision-making. I became familiar with additional frameworks, such as the Ethical Decision-Making Model, which involves identifying the problem, gathering information, identifying options, making a decision, and evaluating the decision. This model provided a structured approach to ethical problem-solving, allowing me to systematically analyse the dilemmas I encountered and make informed decisions.

Moreover, I began engaging in ethical discourse with my colleagues, participating in ethics committees and contributing to scholarly discussions on nursing ethics. These interactions not only expanded my knowledge base but also challenged my own beliefs and biases. They encouraged me to interrogate the underlying assumptions that inform ethical judgements and to consider alternative perspectives.

As I delve into the topic of ethical dilemmas and decision-making in nursing in *The CAR of Nursing*, I aim to shed light on the intricacies of these challenges and provide strategies for navigating through them. I urge nurses to embrace self-reflection, engage in ongoing education and training, and actively participate in ethical discourse. By doing so, we can cultivate a culture of ethical awareness and ensure that our actions uphold the highest standards of integrity and compassion.

Ethical dilemmas are an integral part of nursing practice, and our ability to navigate through them with wisdom and integrity defines our professional identity. It is in the crucible of these challenging moments that the true character of a nurse is revealed. By examining ethical dilemmas faced by nurses and exploring strategies for ethical decision-making, we can equip ourselves with the tools and knowledge necessary to provide the best possible care to our patients, honour their autonomy, and uphold the ethical principles that serve as the cornerstone of our profession.

Speaking up for patients

As I embark upon this chapter, my heart feels heavy with the weight of responsibility. I am reminded of the countless patients I have encountered throughout my career as a nurse, their struggles, their pain, and their vulnerability. It is with a sense of urgency that I address the significance of speaking up for patients and advocating for their needs.

To truly understand the importance of speaking up for our patients, we must first unravel the historical timeline that has led us to where we are today. Throughout the ages, nurses have played a crucial role in caring for the sick and injured. From the days of Florence Nightingale, who revolutionised nursing care during the Crimean War, to the modern era of medical advancements, our profession has always centred on the wellbeing of our patients.

However, in the past, the power dynamics within healthcare systems often marginalised the voices of patients. Doctors held ultimate authority, and nurses were expected to follow orders without question. This hierarchical structure hindered patient-centred care and left patients feeling powerless and unheard.

The CAR of Nursing

It was not until the mid-twentieth century that the concept of patient advocacy started gaining momentum. The civil rights movement and the women's movement paved the way for a shift in societal attitudes, including the advancement of patient rights. As the voice of the patient began to gain recognition, nurses seized the opportunity to step into the role of patient advocate.

The significance of speaking up for patients lies in the fundamental belief that all individuals have the right to be treated with dignity, respect, and appropriate healthcare. As nurses, we have a unique position within the healthcare system, allowing us to bridge the gap between patients and their care providers. We are the ones by their bedside, witnessing their pain, their fears, and their hopes. It is our duty to amplify their voices, to ensure their needs are met, and to advocate for the best possible outcomes.

Patient advocacy encompasses a wide range of responsibilities. It starts with the simple act of listening attentively and empathetically to our patients. By building trust and establishing a therapeutic relationship, we create a safe space for patients to express their concerns and needs. This open communication lays the foundation for effective advocacy.

One important aspect of patient advocacy is ensuring informed consent. Patients have the right to be fully informed about their health conditions, treatment options, and potential risks and benefits. It is our responsibility to provide them with accurate and accessible information, empowering them to make informed decisions about their care.

In addition to ensuring informed consent, advocating for patient safety is paramount. We must be vigilant in identifying and addressing any potential risks or mistakes that may compromise patient wellbeing. This may involve speaking up about medication errors, infections, or inadequate staffing levels. By proactively addressing these concerns, we contribute to creating a culture of safety within our healthcare institutions.

The CAR of Nursing

Another crucial aspect of patient advocacy is addressing disparities in healthcare. Socioeconomic status, race, gender, and other social determinants of health can significantly impact access to quality care. As advocates, we must not only strive to provide equitable care but also challenge systemic barriers and advocate for reforms that promote healthcare justice.

Speaking up for patients also requires collaboration with interdisciplinary teams to ensure coordinated and comprehensive care. By actively participating in care conferences, sharing our expertise, and advocating for the unique needs of our patients, we can contribute to a holistic approach to healthcare.

It is essential to recognise that advocating for patients can sometimes place us in uncomfortable situations. There may be instances where we must challenge the decisions of our superiors, question established protocols, or confront systemic injustices. However, our commitment to our patients should outweigh any personal discomfort. We must be courageous, assertive, and resourceful in our advocacy efforts.

Advocacy should not be confined to the four walls of the hospital or clinic. We must extend our advocacy to the broader community, advocating for public health initiatives, promoting health education, and fighting for policies that prioritise the wellbeing of all individuals. By raising our voices, both individually and collectively, we become agents of change, working towards a healthcare system that truly serves the needs of all.

In conclusion, speaking up for patients and advocating for their needs is not just a responsibility; it is our moral obligation as nurses. By embracing patient advocacy, we have the power to make a profound impact on the lives of those entrusted to our care. Let us never forget the words of Florence Nightingale, who once said, "I attribute my success to this: I never gave or took an excuse." Let us be fearless in our pursuit of justice and unwavering in our commitment to our patients.

The CAR of Nursing

Addressing Healthcare Disparities:

To fully comprehend the scope and magnitude of healthcare disparities, it is essential to understand the historical timeline that has contributed to their existence. This historical timeline traces the roots of healthcare disparities and highlights the key events and milestones that have shaped our current healthcare landscape.

The timeline begins centuries ago, with the colonisation and settlement of different regions across the globe. During this period, Indigenous populations were exposed to new diseases brought by settlers, leading to devastating consequences. The lack of knowledge and resources to combat these diseases further exacerbated healthcare disparities, as Indigenous communities faced disproportionate rates of illness and mortality.

Fast forward to the nineteenth century, a time marked by rapid industrialisation and urbanisation. As cities grew and populations increased, healthcare systems struggled to keep pace with the demands of a rapidly changing society. This era saw the emergence of overcrowded and unsanitary living conditions, which disproportionately impacted marginalised communities. Lack of access to proper sanitation and healthcare services led to higher rates of infectious diseases and poorer health outcomes.

The early twentieth century witnessed significant advancements in healthcare technology and the establishment of formal healthcare systems. Yet, despite these advancements, healthcare disparities persisted, fuelled by a range of factors including socioeconomic status, education, and geographic location. Poverty became a significant determinant of health, as individuals with limited financial resources struggled to access and afford healthcare services. This further deepened the divide between those with access to quality healthcare and those left behind.

It was not until the twenty-first century that a concerted effort began to address healthcare disparities directly. Since then, a growing body of research has revealed the multifaceted nature of healthcare disparities and the role that nurses can play in addressing them. One key area where nurses have emerged as change agents is advocacy. Nurses can leverage their unique position as trusted healthcare providers to advocate for marginalised populations and promote policies that reduce disparities. By addressing social determinants of health, such as poverty, education, and access to healthcare services, nurses can contribute to the dismantling of systemic barriers that perpetuate disparities.

Cultural competence is another critical aspect of nursing practice that can help to bridge the gap in healthcare delivery. As nurses, we must strive to provide culturally competent care to diverse patient populations. This requires an understanding and respect for the unique beliefs, values, and practices of different cultures. By recognising and addressing cultural gaps in healthcare delivery, nurses can ensure that all patients, regardless of their background, receive equitable and high-quality care.

In addition to advocacy and cultural competence, nurses have a vital role to play in health education. In many underserved areas, access to information about preventive measures, healthy lifestyle choices, and disease management is limited. Nurses can fill this gap by actively engaging with patients and communities to provide education and support. By empowering individuals with knowledge, nurses can help communities take charge of their health and bridge the disparities gap.

Furthermore, nurses can foster collaboration among healthcare professionals, community organisations, and policymakers to develop and implement strategies that promote equity in healthcare delivery. By leveraging their interdisciplinary skills and expertise, nurses can contribute to the development of comprehensive solutions that address the multifaceted nature of healthcare disparities. Through collaborative efforts, nurses can help create systemic changes that prioritise equity and ensure that no individual is left behind.

Research and evidence-based practice are also vital tools in the nurse's arsenal when it comes to addressing healthcare disparities. Nurses can actively contribute to research efforts aimed at understanding healthcare disparities and identifying effective interventions to address them. By incorporating evidence-based practices into their care, nurses can help improve health outcomes for all patients, regardless of their social or demographic backgrounds. This commitment to evidence-based practice ensures that healthcare interventions are grounded in scientific research and have been proven effective in reducing disparities.

The role of nurses in addressing healthcare disparities and promoting equity is multifaceted and continues to evolve. As healthcare professionals, we must remain committed to challenging the status quo and advocating for change. By addressing social determinants of health, advocating for policy changes, providing culturally competent care, empowering communities through education, and engaging in collaborative efforts, nurses can make a significant impact in reducing healthcare disparities and promoting equity for all. Through our collective efforts, we can strive for a future where every individual has equal access to healthcare, and no one is left behind.

Policy Advocacy:

As a nurse, I have always believed in the power of policy advocacy to create positive changes in nursing practice and the delivery of patient care. Policy advocacy involves speaking up and taking action to influence health policies at the local, national, and global levels. It is a crucial aspect of nursing that requires nurses to engage in political and legislative processes to advance the interests of patients, healthcare providers, and our profession. In this chapter, we will delve into the impact of policy advocacy on nursing practice and patient care, underscoring its significance and exploring the various ways in which it can be achieved.

The role of policy advocacy in nursing cannot be overstated. Through policy advocacy, nurses can effect systemic changes that address the structural barriers and inequalities in healthcare. By voicing our concerns, promoting evidence-based practices, and engaging in health policy development, we can shape the future of nursing and improve the quality of patient care. Policy advocacy empowers nurses to advocate for their patients' rights, ensure access to quality healthcare, and promote health equity.

One way policy advocacy impacts nursing practice is by influencing the allocation of healthcare resources. Through active engagement in policy development, nurses can advocate for increased funding for healthcare facilities, improved staffing ratios, and the implementation of innovative healthcare programs. These efforts help to ensure that nurses have the necessary resources to provide optimal care. Additionally, policy advocacy can help in securing funding for research and educational initiatives that strengthen nursing practice and improve patient outcomes.

Moreover, policy advocacy plays a crucial role in shaping nursing practice standards. Nurses have a unique perspective on healthcare delivery, and it is through policy advocacy that we can make our voices heard in the development of healthcare policies and regulations. By actively participating in professional organisations, attending conferences, and engaging with policymakers, nurses can advocate for evidence-based practices and standards that align with the needs and best interests of patients. Through policy advocacy, we can advance nursing practice by influencing the creation of policies that support patient-centred care, interdisciplinary collaboration, and continuing education for healthcare professionals.

Policy advocacy also aids in the promotion of health equity. As nurses, we witness firsthand the disparities in healthcare access and outcomes faced by marginalised communities. Through policy advocacy, we can address these disparities by advocating for policies that promote social justice, reduce health inequities, and improve healthcare outcomes for all individuals, regardless of their socioeconomic background or demographic characteristics. This includes advocating for policies that address systemic racism, poverty, and other social determinants of health that contribute to health disparities.

In addition to its impact on nursing practice, policy advocacy directly affects patient care. By advocating for healthcare policies that prioritise patient safety, quality care, and patient rights, nurses can significantly enhance the care they provide. This may include advocating for policies that enforce patient-centred care models, improved patient-staff ratios, and better access to preventive healthcare services. Through policy advocacy, nurses have the power to transform the healthcare system into one that prioritises patient needs, preferences, and outcomes.

Policy advocacy also allows nurses to address the unique healthcare needs of vulnerable populations. By advocating for policies that support the provision of culturally sensitive care, linguistic access, and targeted interventions, nurses can ensure that marginalised populations receive the care they deserve. For example, policy advocacy can involve lobbying for increased funding for programs that provide mental health support for communities affected by trauma or advocating for policies that improve access to healthcare services for individuals with disabilities. These efforts can have a profound impact on the lives of patients, improving their health outcomes and overall wellbeing.

In conclusion, policy advocacy plays a pivotal role in nursing practice and patient care. Through policy advocacy, nurses can shape healthcare policies, influence resource allocation, and promote health equity. By actively engaging in political and legislative processes, nurses can advocate for the needs and rights of their patients, improve nursing practice standards, and enhance the quality of patient care. Policy advocacy is a fundamental aspect of nursing that empowers us to be agents of change, creating a healthcare system that is equitable, accessible, and patient-centred.

Chapter 12:
The Window of Reflection

The Mirror of Self-Awareness:

As a Clinical nurse, I have come to understand that providing compassionate care goes beyond administering medications, dressing wounds, and monitoring vital signs. It requires the ability to connect with patients on a deep and empathetic level, to truly understand their needs and fears, and to provide a safe and nurturing environment for healing. And at the heart of this ability lies self-awareness – the mirror that reflects not only our own internal landscape but also the way in which we perceive and interact with the world around us.

Self-awareness is a concept often overlooked in nursing practice, yet its importance cannot be overstated. When we possess a deep understanding of ourselves, our emotions, and our biases, we are better equipped to provide care that is unbiased, patient-centred, and truly empathetic. It allows us to recognize our strengths and limitations, enabling us to continually improve our skills and knowledge to better serve our patients.

To explore the significance of self-awareness in nursing, we must first understand its essence. Self-awareness encompasses a range of dimensions, including self-reflection, self-regulation, and self-compassion. It involves an honest examination of one's thoughts, feelings, and actions, and the ability to recognize how they influence patient care.

Self-reflection is an integral part of self-awareness in nursing practice. It requires deliberate introspection and a willingness to examine our own biases, beliefs, and values. Through self-reflection, we can identify any preconceived notions or judgments that may affect our ability to provide compassionate care. It allows us to challenge our own assumptions and remain open-minded when interacting with patients from diverse backgrounds and experiences.

In addition to self-awareness, self-regulation is also a crucial element that cannot be overlooked. The skill required for this involves the capability to effectively manage and regulate one's emotions, impulses, and reactions when confronted with difficult circumstances. In our role as nurses, it is not uncommon for us to come across patients who are experiencing pain or distress. Despite the potential emotional hardships, it is of the utmost importance that we make a conscious effort to preserve a sense of calmness and composure. Through the implementation of self-regulation techniques, we are able to uphold a professional demeanour, ensuring that we can offer the essential support and comfort to our patients, all the while ensuring that our own reactions do not impede the quality of their care.

Self-compassion plays a vital role in self-awareness as well. Nursing can be an emotionally demanding profession, and it is easy to become overwhelmed by the suffering we witness daily. It is essential for us to recognize our own emotions and show compassion towards ourselves. By acknowledging our own needs and seeking the support and guidance we require, we can replenish our emotional reserves and continue to provide compassionate care.

Incorporating self-awareness into our nursing practice brings forth a multitude of benefits, both for ourselves and our patients. When nurses are self-aware, they contribute to a culture of safety and open communication within healthcare settings. By recognizing and addressing their own limitations, nurses can effectively collaborate with colleagues, share knowledge, and seek help when needed. They can also demonstrate humility and a willingness to continuously learn, promoting a culture of lifelong learning and professional growth.

In addition, self-aware nurses are better able to establish rapport and build trust with their patients. By understanding their own emotions, nurses can empathize with their patients' fears and concerns, creating an environment that is conducive to healing and recovery. Self-awareness allows nurses to recognize their own biases and prejudices, enabling them to provide equal and unbiased care to all patients, regardless of their race, gender, or social status.

Furthermore, self-awareness enhances communication skills in nursing practice. Nurses who are aware of their own communication styles can adapt their approach to effectively communicate with patients and their families. By being present in the moment and actively listening to their patients, nurses can better understand their needs and concerns, leading to improved patient outcomes and satisfaction.

Self-awareness also contributes to the prevention of burnout and compassion fatigue, two common challenges faced by healthcare professionals. By recognising the signs of emotional exhaustion and taking proactive steps to address it, nurses can protect their own wellbeing and ensure their ability to provide high-quality care over the long term. Self-awareness helps nurses set boundaries, engage in self-care practices, and seek support when needed, ultimately promoting their own resilience and preventing burnout.

In conclusion, self-awareness is an essential aspect of nursing practice that should not be underestimated. By exploring and nurturing our own self-awareness, we can provide compassionate care that is unbiased, patient-centred, and empathetic. Self-reflection, self-regulation, and self-compassion serve as the foundations for this journey of self-awareness, enabling us to continuously grow, learn, and adapt in our nursing practice. By embracing self-awareness, we can truly become the mirrors that reflect the compassion and care that our patients deserve.

The Pond of Mindfulness:

Whenever I enter the peaceful and calm realm of nursing, I am consistently reminded of how crucial it is to be present and attentive in the care we offer our patients. Throughout my personal journey of pursuing a career in nursing, I have gained a profound understanding that being fully present, both in body and mind, extends not only to the well-being of our patients but also to our own personal fulfilment. This understanding has sparked my curiosity to delve into the concept of mindfulness and its practicality in the nursing profession.

The CAR of Nursing

Mindfulness, as defined by Jon Kabat-Zinn, is the practice of paying attention in a particular way: on purpose, in the present moment, and non-judgmentally. It is the act of being fully aware of one's thoughts, emotions, and sensations in the present moment, without getting caught up in judgments or distractions. While mindfulness has gained popularity in recent years, its roots can be traced back to ancient contemplative traditions such as Buddhism.

In the context of nursing, mindfulness serves as a powerful tool to enhance presence and attentiveness in patient care. By cultivating mindfulness, nurses can develop a deep understanding of their patients' needs and experiences, allowing for a more compassionate and holistic approach to their care. As I delve deeper into the pond of mindfulness, I am amazed at the multitude of ways in which it can be integrated into our practice.

One of the primary applications of mindfulness in nursing is the development of self-awareness. By cultivating mindfulness, nurses can become more attuned to their own thoughts, emotions, and physical sensations, and the impact they have on their interactions with patients. This self-awareness serves as a foundation for cultivating empathy and compassion—an essential aspect of nursing. By being fully present and non-judgmental, nurses can create a safe and supportive environment for their patients, where they feel heard and understood.

Moreover, mindfulness can enhance nurses' ability to manage stress and prevent burnout—a significant issue in the nursing profession. The demanding and often emotionally charged nature of our work can take a toll on our mental and physical wellbeing. By incorporating mindfulness practices such as meditation and deep breathing into our daily routines, nurses can develop resilience and cope more effectively with stress. Mindfulness allows us to step back from the chaos and demands of the job, centre ourselves in the present moment, and find balance amidst the challenges.

In addition to these personal benefits, mindfulness can also improve patient outcomes. Numerous studies have shown that mindfulness-based interventions can reduce symptoms of anxiety and depression, improve pain management, and enhance overall wellbeing in patients. By incorporating mindfulness techniques into our care, such as guided imagery, deep breathing exercises, and body scan meditations, nurses can empower their patients to take an active role in their healing process. Mindful practices not only help patients manage their symptoms but also foster a sense of control and self-efficacy, ensuring a more satisfying healthcare experience.

Nursing education also stands to benefit from the integration of mindfulness. By incorporating mindfulness training into nursing curricula, aspiring nurses can develop the skills to navigate the increasingly complex and fast-paced world of healthcare. Mindfulness-based stress reduction programs, for example, can equip nurses with coping strategies that they can utilise throughout their careers. Furthermore, mindfulness can foster critical thinking and clinical judgement, allowing nurses to approach patient care with a sense of curiosity and open-mindedness.

The pond of mindfulness is vast and ever-expanding. As I continue to explore its depths, I am humbled by its transformative power in nursing. Mindfulness has the potential to revolutionise the way we care for our patients and ourselves. By cultivating presence and attentiveness through mindfulness, we can create a ripple effect, touching the lives of those in our care and in our profession. The journey into the pond of mindfulness is not without its challenges, but the rewards are immeasurable, both for nurses and their patients. Let us dive in together and embrace the transformative power of mindfulness in the sacred art of nursing.

The Gallery of Lessons Learned:

The walls are adorned with framed stories, each one meticulously curated to highlight the triumphs and trials in the journey of nursing. Each story represents a unique lesson learned, a pivotal moment that has shaped the trajectory of countless nurses' lives and improved patient outcomes. As I walk through the gallery, I can't help but be struck by the diversity of experiences and the wealth of knowledge encapsulated within each frame.

Amidst all the stories, one in particular captured my attention with its vibrant colours and hauntingly captivating narrative. A nurse is confronted with a challenging ethical dilemma, leading her to confront her own biases and prejudices. Maria, a nurse in this scenario, faced an ethical dilemma: should she prioritise the patient's religious beliefs, resulting in their rejection of blood transfusions, or should she take assertive action against their wishes to ensure their survival?

Maria's story delves into the emotional turmoil she experienced as she grappled with the weight of her decision. The framed narrative offers a glimpse into the world of moral distress and ethical dilemmas that nurses often face, reminding us of the delicate balance between respecting autonomy and advocating for the best interests of the patient.

As I read Maria's story, I am struck by the courage and humility she demonstrated by sharing her mistake. Maria acknowledges that she initially allowed her personal beliefs to cloud her judgement, causing her to dismiss the patient's wishes without truly understanding their cultural and religious context. By acknowledging her mistake, Maria opens herself up to growth and learning, paving the way for other nurses to better navigate similar situations in the future.

The gallery also features research studies that further enlighten me on the importance of reflecting on past experiences and mistakes. One study, conducted by Johnson and colleagues, explores the impact of nurses' reflection on patient safety incidents. The researchers found that nurses who engaged in structured reflection on past incidents were more likely to identify root causes, develop strategies for improvement, and prevent similar incidents from occurring in the future.

This observation aligns with another study by Ramirez and co-authors, which examines the concept of the "wisdom of hindsight" in the nursing profession. The researchers highlight how reflecting on past experiences can enhance professional judgement and decision-making, ultimately leading to better patient outcomes. Nurses who take the time to learn from their mistakes and critically examine their own practice are better equipped to provide safe, efficient, and compassionate care.

Walking deeper into the gallery, I stumble upon a section dedicated to personal narratives written by nurses from different specialties and backgrounds. These narratives offer a raw and unfiltered glimpse into the realities of nursing, highlighting the challenges, failures, and triumphs that define the profession. Reading these stories, I am reminded of the importance of creating a culture that encourages nurses to openly discuss and learn from their mistakes.

In one poignant tale, a nurse recounts the pain of losing a patient due to a medication error. The nurse, overwhelmed with guilt and self-doubt, shares how this devastating event served as a catalyst for change in her practice. She enrolled in medication safety courses, implemented double-check protocols, and dedicated herself to thorough documentation and vigilance. Through sharing her story, she hopes to inspire others to prioritise patient safety and learn from her own painful experience.

The Gallery of Lessons Learned serves as a powerful reminder of the value of reflection and growth in nursing practice. It invites nurses from all walks of life to embrace their mistakes, to learn from them, and to transform their actions into meaningful change. In this hallowed space, past experiences become powerful beacons of light, guiding us towards improved patient outcomes and a more compassionate and competent nursing profession.

As I exit the gallery, a renewed sense of purpose fills my heart. The stories I encountered within those walls have left an indelible mark on my soul. I am reminded of the immense responsibility we carry as nurses, but also the immense power we possess to make a difference. The Gallery of Lessons Learned stands as a testament to the transformative potential of humility, reflection, and growth. It is a reminder that our past experiences and mistakes, when embraced and understood, can shape us into better caregivers, advocates, and healers.

I leave the gallery, humbled and inspired, ready to embrace the lessons of the past and forge a new path towards excellence in nursing practice.

Chapter 13:
The Seat Belt of Safety

Patient safety in healthcare:

As one of the hand hygiene auditors in my workplace, I firmly believe that it would be a grave mistake to neglect patient safety when writing about the core of nursing. Patient safety encompasses more than just the prevention of accidents or mishaps; it is a comprehensive approach to ensuring the well-being and security of patients. The first point to consider is the establishment of a culture of safety within healthcare organisations. The aim is to create a setting where each team member is empowered and acknowledges their responsibility in maintaining patient safety. The primary goal is to promote the development of open communication, respect, and collaboration among all healthcare providers, including nurses, doctors, and support staff. By collaborating, actively exchanging information, and ensuring each other's well-being, we can significantly reduce the potential hazards that our patients may face.

Implementing evidence-based practices is another vital aspect of ensuring patient safety. Research-driven guidelines and protocols have transformed healthcare by providing healthcare professionals with a robust foundation for decision-making. Evidence-based practices improve patient outcomes, reduce unnecessary interventions, and promote efficient resource allocation. By adhering to evidence-based practices, we can minimise the likelihood of errors, enhance patient care, and ultimately save lives.

One of the primary goals of patient safety is to reduce medical errors. These errors can occur at any level of the healthcare system, from diagnosis and treatment to medication administration and discharge planning. Reducing medical errors requires constant vigilance, attention to detail, and ongoing improvement in our healthcare processes. Identifying and addressing systemic shortcomings that contribute to errors, such as a lack of standardised practices, inadequate communication, or reliance on memory rather than written protocols, is crucial. By proactively identifying and rectifying these issues, we can prevent potentially catastrophic consequences for our patients.

The impact of patient safety on healthcare outcomes cannot be overstated. When patient safety is prioritised, healthcare organisations see a substantial reduction in mortality rates. Lives that could have been lost due to medical errors or preventable mishaps are saved, and families are spared the devastating grief of losing a loved one prematurely. Moreover, patient safety initiatives lead to a significant decrease in hospital-acquired infections. By implementing strict infection control practices, adhering to hand hygiene protocols, and meticulously maintaining a sterile environment, we can prevent the spread of dangerous pathogens and safeguard the health of our patients.

Patient safety is also instrumental in enhancing patient satisfaction with the healthcare experience. When patients feel safe and well-cared for, their overall satisfaction increases. They are more likely to trust their healthcare providers, cooperate with treatment plans, and have a positive outlook on their recovery journey. Conversely, when patient safety is compromised, patient satisfaction plummets. This can lead to disillusionment, fear, and a loss of confidence in the healthcare system. Therefore, it is crucial to prioritise patient safety to not only improve medical outcomes but also foster a positive and trusting relationship between patients and their healthcare providers.

Beyond individual patient outcomes, patient safety initiatives also have a profound impact on the healthcare system. For instance, they help reduce healthcare costs associated with preventable errors or adverse events. The financial burden of medical errors is substantial, often resulting in prolonged hospital stays, additional treatments, and legal consequences. By systematically addressing patient safety concerns, healthcare organisations can mitigate these unnecessary costs, ultimately benefiting both patients and the healthcare system at large.

In conclusion, patient safety in healthcare is of utmost importance. It represents our unwavering commitment to protect and care for our patients, advocating for their wellbeing above all else. By fostering a culture of safety, implementing evidence-based practices, and proactively addressing medical errors, we can substantially improve healthcare outcomes. Patient safety saves lives, reduces hospital-acquired infections, enhances patient satisfaction, and ultimately fosters trust in the healthcare system. As nurses, we must be acutely aware of the impact of patient safety and work tirelessly to ensure the safety of our patients. It is both a professional and moral imperative, underscoring the core values of nursing and the essence of our noble profession.

Preventing medical errors:

Throughout my extensive years of experience in the nursing field, I have come to deeply understand the importance of adopting a comprehensive approach to prevent medical errors. It begins with a strong foundation of knowledge and understanding of the potential risks and vulnerabilities in healthcare settings. By staying informed about the latest research and evidence-based practices, I am better equipped to identify and proactively address potential areas of concern.

One strategy that I find particularly effective in preventing medical errors is implementing a robust medication administration system. This system includes several checks and balances to ensure that the right medication is given in the correct dosage, to the right patient, at the right time. It starts with verifying the medication orders, double-checking the patient's identity, and calculating and measuring the accurate dose. Before administration, I always take a moment to review any potential drug interactions or contraindications, considering the patient's current condition and medical history. This thorough process significantly reduces the risk of medication errors, ensuring patient safety.

Another aspect of preventing medical errors that cannot be overlooked is effective communication. In a healthcare team, open and transparent communication is essential for ensuring that everyone is on the same page and working towards a common goal – the well-being of the patient. By actively listening to colleagues and other healthcare providers, we can catch any misunderstandings or discrepancies that may lead to errors. Additionally, clear and concise documentation is crucial in transferring information accurately between shifts, preventing any breakdown in continuity of care. As a nurse, I make it a priority to communicate clearly and effectively, ensuring that all necessary information is conveyed accurately to the appropriate parties.

Equally important in preventing medical errors is the implementation of best practices and adherence to evidence-based guidelines. By following well-established protocols, such as hand hygiene, standard precautions, and proper documentation, we can minimise the risk of errors and ensure consistent, high-quality care. Regularly reviewing and updating these best practices based on new research and guidelines is essential to keep up with advancements in healthcare and provide the best possible care to our patients.

While individual efforts are critical in preventing medical errors, fostering a culture of safety within healthcare organisations is equally vital. This culture emphasises the importance of reporting errors or near misses without fear of blame or punishment, encouraging a focus on learning and improvement rather than retribution. By creating an environment where errors are viewed as opportunities to identify system weaknesses and improve patient safety, we can collectively work towards preventing future errors. This culture of safety also extends to the encouragement of interdisciplinary collaboration and support, recognising that each healthcare professional brings a unique perspective and expertise to the table.

In summary, preventing medical errors requires a multifaceted approach that starts with a strong knowledge base and understanding of potential risks. By implementing robust medication administration systems, ensuring effective communication, adhering to evidence-based guidelines, and fostering a culture of safety, we can significantly reduce the risk of errors and ensure patient safety. As a nurse, I am committed to continually improving my practice and actively seeking ways to prevent medical errors to provide the highest quality of care to my patients.

Infection control and safety protocols:

First and foremost, hand hygiene stands as the foundation of infection control. Regular handwashing or using hand sanitisers can significantly reduce the transmission of pathogens. By maintaining proper hand hygiene, healthcare workers break the cycle of contamination and prevent the spread of potentially harmful microorganisms. It is not just a routine chore but a fundamental responsibility. Patients, healthcare workers, and visitors alike must understand the importance of this simple act, as it can truly save lives.

In addition to hand hygiene, the use of personal protective equipment (PPE) is crucial in ensuring the safety of all individuals involved in healthcare settings. Gloves, masks, gowns, and other protective gear form a vital barrier between healthcare workers and infectious agents, minimising the risk of exposure. Understanding the appropriate use of PPE and diligently following protocols is essential for healthcare professionals, as it safeguards their health while they care for others.

Proper waste management is another crucial aspect of infection control and safety protocols. Disposing of medical waste, sharps, and hazardous materials appropriately is imperative to prevent contamination and reduce the risk of injuries. Mishandling or improper disposal of these items can have severe consequences, both for the individuals directly involved and for the wider healthcare environment. Ensuring that waste management protocols are strictly followed is paramount to maintaining a safe and clean healthcare environment.

Sterilisation and disinfection are essential practices in healthcare settings. Medical equipment must be thoroughly sterilised to eliminate any potential pathogens. Surfaces and patient areas also need regular disinfection to minimise the risk of contamination. These processes are meticulous and require adherence to industry-standard procedures. Only through proper sterilisation and disinfection can we provide a safe and sterile environment for patients, minimising the risk of healthcare-associated infections.

Isolation precautions play a vital role in preventing the spread of infections. Different types of isolation precautions, such as contact, droplet, and airborne precautions, are implemented based on the specific infectious agents. Patients with highly contagious illnesses are isolated to limit their contact with others, preventing the transmission of infectious diseases. These precautions are crucial not only for the infected individuals but also for the protection of other patients, healthcare workers, and visitors.

Vaccination is a cornerstone of infection control, providing protection against vaccine-preventable diseases. It is essential for healthcare workers to maintain up-to-date immunisations to safeguard themselves, their patients, and the broader community. By being immunised, healthcare professionals can significantly reduce the risk of contracting or spreading infectious diseases, thereby promoting a safe and healthy healthcare environment.

The importance of maintaining a clean and safe healthcare environment cannot be overstated. Proper ventilation, air filtration, and regular cleaning and disinfection are all essential components of maintaining a healthy environment. A well-maintained healthcare environment not only contributes to the prevention of infections but also creates a favourable healing environment for patients. Cleanliness and hygiene must be regarded as non-negotiable aspects of healthcare.

Education and training are crucial for healthcare workers to understand and implement infection control practices and safety protocols. Continuous education and training programs ensure that healthcare professionals stay updated with the latest guidelines and best practices. It is essential to foster a culture of learning and professional growth, as it directly influences the quality and safety of patient care. Through comprehensive education and training, healthcare workers can acquire the necessary knowledge and skills to navigate the complex landscape of infection control.

Surveillance and monitoring systems play a crucial role in identifying and responding to potential outbreaks or infections. These systems enable healthcare organisations to track the occurrence and transmission of infectious diseases, facilitating prompt intervention and control measures. Monitoring compliance with infection control measures ensures that healthcare professionals are adhering to the established protocols and guidelines, further enhancing the safety of patients and healthcare workers.

Effective communication and collaboration are vital for successful infection control and the enforcement of safety protocols. Clear and concise communication among healthcare teams, patients, and visitors fosters a shared understanding of the importance of infection control measures. Collaboration promotes adherence to protocols and enhances overall safety within the healthcare environment. By working together, we create a supportive and safe atmosphere that prioritises the well-being of all individuals involved.

In conclusion, infection control measures and safety protocols are the very backbone of healthcare settings. They are not mere formalities; they are vital to prevent the spread of infections and safeguard the well-being of patients, healthcare workers, and visitors. Through hand hygiene, the use of personal protective equipment, proper waste management, sterilisation and disinfection, isolation precautions, vaccination, environmental controls, education and training, surveillance and monitoring, and effective collaboration and communication, we can create a healthcare environment that is safe, clean, and conducive to healing. By embracing these practices and protocols, we uphold our commitment to providing the highest standards of care to those who rely on us.

Creating a culture of safety:

Research has highlighted the significance of organisational culture in ensuring and enhancing patient safety. The studies emphasise that a culture of safety is not simply a nice-to-have but a fundamental necessity. It goes beyond policies and procedures to create an environment where safety is ingrained in every action, decision, and interaction.

Effective leadership is a key driver in fostering a culture of safety. Leaders who prioritise safety and model safe behaviours set the tone for the entire organisation. When leaders consistently demonstrate a commitment to safety, it sends a clear message to all staff members that safety is not negotiable. Safety is not just a box to be ticked but an ethos that permeates every aspect of care delivery.

Clear communication plays an integral role in promoting a culture of safety. In a fast-paced and high-stress environment like healthcare, effective communication ensures that essential information is relayed accurately, timely, and without ambiguity. This is vital not only for smooth workflow but also for identifying and addressing potential safety concerns. Communication breakdowns have been identified as a leading cause of adverse events, so it is imperative to foster an environment where open and honest communication is encouraged.

Engaging all stakeholders in safety initiatives is crucial for the success of a culture of safety. This includes not only healthcare professionals but also patients and their families. Patients should feel empowered to actively participate in their own care, while their families should be involved as partners in the journey to ensure their loved ones' safety. By involving all stakeholders, a sense of shared responsibility and collective accountability is fostered, leading to a safer healthcare environment.

Continuous learning is a cornerstone of a culture of safety. It is essential to create an environment that encourages healthcare professionals to engage in lifelong learning and professional development. This includes staying up to date with evidence-based practices, attending educational programs, and participating in quality improvement initiatives. By continuously seeking knowledge and improvement, healthcare professionals demonstrate a commitment to providing the highest level of safe and effective care to their patients.

Feedback, both positive and constructive, is essential for fostering a culture of safety. Feedback provides an opportunity for individuals and teams to reflect on their performance, identify areas for improvement, and celebrate successes. Feedback should be given in a timely and respectful manner, focusing on learning and growth rather than blame or punishment. By creating an environment where feedback is valued and encouraged, healthcare professionals are empowered to continuously improve their practice and contribute to a safer healthcare environment.

Implementing strategies and best practices is vital for creating a culture of safety in nursing and healthcare settings. Organisations should establish systems and processes that support safety, such as incident reporting, medication reconciliation, and effective handoff communication. Regular safety audits and assessments should be conducted to identify potential risks and areas for improvement. Investing in resources and technologies that enhance safety, such as electronic health records and barcode medication administration, can also contribute to a safer healthcare environment.

In conclusion, organisational culture plays a critical role in promoting a safe healthcare environment. By prioritising safety, fostering effective leadership, promoting clear communication, engaging all stakeholders, emphasising continuous learning and improvement, and implementing best practices, a culture of safety can be established and nurtured. It is through these collective efforts that nursing and healthcare organisations can create an environment where patients and healthcare professionals feel safe, supported, and confident in the care provided.

Patient advocacy for safety:

In the world of healthcare, patient safety is of paramount importance. Advocating for the safety of patients is not only a professional responsibility but also a moral duty that every nurse must uphold. As a nurse, I have dedicated my life to caring for others, and within the realm of patient advocacy, my ultimate goal is to empower readers to become advocates for patient safety and encourage proactive measures. In this chapter, we explore the critical aspects of patient advocacy for safety, its significance, challenges, and the essential strategies that every nurse and healthcare professional must embrace.

Patient safety is not a topic to be taken lightly; it is a matter of life or death. Every day, healthcare facilities are faced with the daunting task of providing care for patients who entrust their lives to us. Yet, despite the best intentions and efforts, medical errors and adverse events continue to occur, often at a staggering rate. It is estimated that medical errors are responsible for approximately 250,000 deaths in the United States each year, making it the third leading cause of death in the country (Makary & Daniel, 2016). These statistics are alarming and highlight the urgent need for patient advocacy.

We can prevent or reduce this by using the acronym CAR. If you are concerned about a patient or a family member, take action. Even if you think you might be wrong, let the person know what you are concerned about by following the three letters of CAR: What are you concerned about? What is your action? What is the result? By completing these three steps every time, we can recognise a problem and take action to reduce its occurrence, thereby minimising incidents that lead to regret or self-blame.

It is essential to recognise that advocacy for patient safety is not limited to healthcare professionals alone; it requires the collective effort of all stakeholders, including patients and their families. Readers must become informed advocates capable of identifying potential risks, speaking up on behalf of patients, and actively engaging in preventive measures that ensure their safety.

To fulfil our role as advocates for patient safety, we must first acknowledge the challenges that hinder our progress. One such challenge is the hierarchical nature of healthcare systems, where power dynamics often discourage open communication and the voicing of concerns. The perceived authority of physicians and senior healthcare professionals can create an environment where subordinates feel hesitant to challenge decisions. However, it is imperative to overcome these barriers and foster a culture of open dialogue and collaboration, where all members of the healthcare team have a voice and are empowered to speak up when patient safety is at risk.

Furthermore, healthcare professionals must navigate the intricate landscape of misinformation and medical complexities. Rapid advancements in technology and treatment modalities can sometimes lead to confusion and lapses in patient safety. In an era of information overload, it is essential for healthcare professionals to stay up to date with evidence-based practices, research, and guidelines. By continually expanding our knowledge and embracing lifelong learning, we equip ourselves with the necessary tools to advocate effectively for patient safety.

In addition to personal and professional growth, integrating technology in healthcare has the potential to revolutionise patient safety. Electronic Health Records (EHR), medication administration systems, and patient monitoring devices enable us to track and analyse patient data in real time, facilitating early identification and intervention in potential safety risks. Embracing technology also means investing in infrastructure and staff training to ensure seamless integration into the healthcare environment. As a writer, I encourage you to learn, adapt, and advocate for implementing technology-driven solutions that enhance patient safety.

While technological advancements are pivotal, we must not overlook the significance of compassionate and patient-centred care. Beyond physical safety, emotional and psychological well-being are essential components of patient safety. It is crucial for healthcare professionals to actively listen to patients, acknowledge their fears and concerns, and provide holistic care that goes beyond the disease or condition being treated. Empathy and compassion are intrinsic qualities that nurture trust and contribute to a safer healthcare experience for patients.

Nurse empowerment is another critical factor in patient advocacy for safety. As nurses, we are the frontline caregivers, spending the most time with patients and intimately understanding their needs. Therefore, nursing leaders and organisations need to invest in the professional development of nurses, providing them with the necessary resources, education, and opportunities to grow and make a significant impact on patient safety. By empowering nurses, we empower the entire healthcare system to prioritise patient safety and advocate for change.

In conclusion, patient advocacy for safety is a complex and multifaceted endeavour that demands the commitment and dedication of all healthcare stakeholders. Through our journey together in this book, my aim is not only to educate and inform but also to inspire you to take an active role in advocating for patient safety. By embracing a proactive approach, overcoming challenges, and remaining steadfast in our pursuit of excellence, we can create a culture of patient safety that ensures the well-being of every individual under our care. Together, let us become the driving force behind a healthcare system that prioritises patient safety.

Chapter 14:
The Seat Of Holistic Healthcare Delivery

The successful completion of this book can largely be attributed to a thorough exploration of the fundamental principles that underpin holistic healthcare delivery. To deliver effective holistic care, it is essential to embrace a comprehensive approach that encompasses various dimensions of well-being. This requires careful attention to every aspect of care, ensuring that no detail goes unnoticed. It is also crucial to acknowledge the range of challenges that come with holistic healthcare, as these obstacles are significant and should not be underestimated.

Through 15 years of nursing and observational research, I came to recognise five key elements of human needs essential for providing holistic care. These elements, known as PSEMS, refer to Physical, Social, Emotional, Mental, and Spiritual needs. Healthcare providers, no matter where they are or the context in which they work, should adhere to a cohesive framework that fosters optimal utilisation and effectiveness of care. Consistency in practice is vital for delivering high-quality healthcare that meets individuals' needs and ultimately helps reduce hospital and care facility readmissions. Before anyone is discharged from a hospital or a care facility, it is imperative that the care provider examines all letters of PSEMS. The order in which these needs are addressed does not matter; the urgency of each depends on the healthcare provider concerned.

Let us examine each component of PSEMS in greater detail. Understanding these facets is fundamental to delivering comprehensive, holistic care that meets patients' diverse needs.

The P stands for Physical need. What is their complaint? People need to communicate the reasons for their admission to effectively address their physical needs. Do they need essential medical treatments, such as oxygen therapy, blood transfusions, or other critical interventions? These points highlight the importance of addressing physical needs. Establishing a consistent and comfortable routine, which includes regular waste elimination, plays a significant role in meeting these needs. Good hygiene practices are also essential, as they help prevent infections and create a clean, pleasant environment for recovery. Effectively managing and alleviating pain stands at the forefront of physical care needs, aiming to enhance comfort and support a quicker recovery.

Furthermore, physical care needs do not only apply to healthcare settings. Partners at home should meet various essential physical needs to maintain their well-being and strengthen their relationship. One key need is access to healthy, balanced meals, which are vital to overall health and nutrition. Staying well hydrated is equally essential, meaning you must drink enough water to keep your body functioning optimally. Both partners should prioritise getting enough rest and sleep to ensure they have the energy to tackle daily challenges.

Physical contact—such as hugging, cuddling, holding hands, and kissing—significantly boosts emotional connections between partners. Physical activities can also keep you fit and alleviate stress, whether alone or together. Carving out dedicated time and creating a welcoming atmosphere for both individuals to unwind and recharge is essential, recognising the importance of personal space.

Lastly, ensuring a comfortable living environment is crucial. This involves addressing the needs of both partners, particularly their sense of safety and security in their homes.

Are there any physical needs in your relationship with your partner, family, or work colleague? The CAR approach discussed in the previous chapters can effectively address these concerns. Here are a few examples to help you get started:

1. Step one is openly communicating concerns with your partner, family, or colleague. Share your thoughts on any physical needs you believe are not being fulfilled and communicate your feelings and expectations.
2. Once you have voiced your concerns, it is essential to follow through with action. This might mean establishing limits,

reevaluating roles, or reaching agreements that meet both parties' physical needs.

3. The aim is to achieve a positive result that satisfies your physical needs. This might include better communication, a deeper understanding of each other's needs, and finding solutions that benefit both parties.

By implementing the CAR approach, you can ensure that your physical needs are acknowledged, addressed, and satisfied in any area of your life where issues may emerge. To maintain a healthy relationship or work dynamic, it is crucial always to remember the significance of maintaining open lines of communication, taking proactive measures, and striving for positive results.

The S stands for Social need:

The importance of social needs cannot be overstated for individuals, families, and society. Do not overlook the social needs of those you care for, whether patients, family members, children, or pets.

Social needs are fundamental for human beings as they contribute to our overall well-being and quality of life. It is vital to recognise and address individuals' social needs, as neglecting them can have significant adverse effects on their mental and emotional health.

Social interaction is crucial in patients' recovery and overall treatment outcomes. Connecting with others, whether fellow patients or healthcare providers, helps alleviate feelings of isolation and can provide a support network that aids healing. Social connections offer emotional support, assisting individuals in coping with stress, anxiety, and other mental health challenges. Discharging patients or clients from any care facility should include attention to their social needs.

Similarly, families thrive on social connections. Nurturing relationships with loved ones promotes a sense of belonging, enhances emotional bonds, and fosters a supportive environment. Neglecting social needs within a family unit can lead to strained relationships, increased stress levels, and dissatisfaction.

Children also require social interaction to develop essential social skills, emotional intelligence, and a sense of identity. Engaging in playdates, extracurricular activities, and spending quality time with peers and family members is crucial for their social and emotional development.

Even pets benefit from social interaction. Animals thrive when they have regular contact with their owners and other animals, particularly domesticated ones. This interaction helps prevent loneliness, reduces anxiety, and contributes to their well-being.

Fulfilling social needs is essential for building strong communities and fostering a sense of belonging and unity in broader society. Social connections enable individuals to share experiences, support one another, and contribute positively to their surroundings. Neglecting social needs can lead to social isolation, increased rates of mental health issues, and a breakdown of social cohesion.

These tips can help enhance your social skills:

Remember the significance of your body language, as it can greatly influence the way others perceive you. To communicate engagement effectively, maintain an open posture and avoid crossing your arms; however, this may be normal in other cultures. Use appropriate gestures. Summarise and repeat what the other person has said to ensure you understand them correctly. It is essential to demonstrate empathy and understanding by acknowledging and validating their feelings and experiences, regardless of whether you share the same perspective.

In social situations, initiate conversations with light-hearted topics and gradually delve into more profound subjects. Share personal stories and experiences to build rapport and connect with others. Be mindful of the overall atmosphere of the conversation and adjust your facial expressions accordingly. It is important to practice regularly to improve your social skills. Plan and prepare for social interactions by thinking of topics or questions to keep the conversation flowing smoothly. After each interaction, take a moment to reflect and identify areas for improvement in future encounters. Observe how others interact and learn from social norms and cues.

To expand your social circle, seek out like-minded individuals by joining social groups or participating in activities that align with your interests. Volunteer work enables social interaction and helps develop essential social skills.

Seek feedback from trusted friends or family members on enhancing your social skills. Constructive criticism can be valuable in bringing about positive change. Remember that developing better social skills takes time and patience. Stay resilient and continue practising, as setbacks should not define you. Gradually, you will notice progress if you remain consistent in your efforts.

In conclusion, recognising and addressing social needs is paramount for individuals, families, and society. By prioritising social interactions and fostering strong social connections, we can enhance the well-being and happiness of those we care for and contribute to building a more compassionate and inclusive world.

For society:

Social needs foster social cohesion, creating a more connected and harmonious society. Strong social networks can lead to economic benefits through collaboration, networking, and community support. Societies with strong social bonds tend to have better public health outcomes. Social support can reduce the incidence of mental health issues and chronic diseases. Meeting social needs is fundamental to the well-being and functioning of individuals, families, and society.

How do you see social needs impacting your own life?

When I relocated to Australia in 2007, I found myself in a foreign landscape, unfamiliar and daunting. In those early days, I craved social support to help me navigate this new chapter of my life. I eagerly joined a vibrant community social group, attended a welcoming local church, and engaged with social networking platforms like International. Through these avenues, I gradually connected with a diverse array of individuals from various countries and cultures, each with their unique stories to share.

Having cultivated a robust social network has provided me with an invaluable sense of belonging and emotional support. It is not just about having friends; it is about forging connections that allow me to truly identify with others, share personal experiences, and seek guidance when faced with life's inevitable challenges. This web of relationships has significantly enhanced my emotional well-being, acting as a soothing balm during stressful times and helping to alleviate lingering anxiety.

Moreover, fulfilling my social needs has opened doors for collaboration and networking that I might not have explored otherwise. These interpersonal connections have illuminated new opportunities for both personal and professional growth. Through exchanges of knowledge, skills, and resources, I have not only expanded my horizons but also reaped economic benefits, such as discovering job openings, receiving generous recommendations, and tapping into new markets. Each relationship enriches my life, reinforcing the profound impact that social needs can have on our journey.

Take a moment to reflect on your social needs. If you cannot find an existing group or community that resonates with you, consider creating one yourself. This could be a vibrant group exercise class filled with encouraging participants, an engaging book club where literature is passionately discussed, or a friendly community group where connections can flourish. Even cultivating relationships with work colleagues can provide invaluable support. A strong network of social support enhances your sense of belonging and plays a crucial role in safeguarding your mental well-being. Research shows that nurturing these connections can significantly lower the risk of developing mental health challenges, such as depression and anxiety, while also reducing the likelihood of chronic illnesses like heart disease and diabetes. Embrace the opportunity to foster meaningful relationships; they are vital to a fulfilling and healthy life.

The E stands for Emotional needs:

Our well-being is intricately woven into the fabric of our emotional needs, which make us feel valued, secure, and deeply connected to others. Consider the poignant story of Mrs Saye, a gentle soul in her late 70s who found herself in a new chapter of life after the profound loss of her husband, a partnership that had spanned an incredible 40 years. Although her physical health remained stable, a noticeable pallor had settled over her spirit; she appeared withdrawn and quiet, spending countless hours gazing out the window at the world passing by or sitting alone in the lounge, lost in thought.

The attentive staff quickly recognised that while her basic requirements—food, medication, and safety—were diligently met, an intangible element was absent from her care: a sense of joy and engagement. Among them was Nurse Alexandra, who felt a spark of compassion ignite within her. Instead of adhering strictly to routines, she opted for a more personal approach. With warmth and patience, she encouraged Mrs Saye to share tales from her past, gently drawing her out of her shell as they conversed.

As Mrs Saye opened up, she fondly recalled memories of her husband, their adventures in farming in the sun-drenched landscapes of Africa, and the vibrant crops that danced in the breeze. It was during these conversations that Alexandra discovered Mrs Saye's deep yearning for her beloved garden—a sanctuary that had bestowed her with comfort and purpose for decades.

Motivated by this newfound understanding, Alexandra collaborated with the care team to transform a quiet courtyard corner into a miniature gardening haven. They sourced pots, soil, and a delightful array of flowers, including the very crops that Mrs Saye cherished. Invited to roll up her sleeves and partake in the planting, Mrs Saye's eyes lit up with a glimmer of excitement—a spark that had long been dimmed.

Gradually, the once-quiet woman began to shed her solitude, venturing outdoors and relaxing among colourful blooms and earthy scents. As fellow residents gathered around, drawn by her gardening expertise and kind spirit, laughter and chatter flowed, creating connections that warmed her heart.

By addressing her profound need for purpose and companionship, Mrs Saye's quality of life blossomed in ways the staff had never anticipated. They learned that tending to emotional well-being is just as essential as caring for physical health—nurturing the heart and spirit can lead to true healing and fulfilment.

Let us delve into the heartfelt story of Ms Jones, a spirited 66-year-old resident of our rehabilitation and acute stroke unit. She had been a valued patient for many weeks. I vividly remember one particular Christmas day when I found myself on duty, surrounded by the joyful hum of the holiday spirit that filled the hospital. In an effort to bring comfort and cheer to our patients, the hospital had arranged for everyone to enjoy a festive meal of their choice, ensuring that no one would feel alone on this special day.

As I wandered through the wards, I noticed that all the mobile patients were gathered in the dining room, sharing laughter and memories over their holiday dinners. But Ms Jones, with her trusty wheelie walker by her side, had chosen solitude and refused to join the others. The nursing staff informed me of her decision, and with a sense of concern, I made my way to her room to check on her.

Upon entering, I found Ms Jones reclined on her bed, her meal untouched on the table beside her. The vibrant colours of the holiday feast seemed to pale in comparison to the despondent look on her face. I approached her gently and inquired about the root of her sadness, asking if she was in any discomfort. She shook her head, but her eyes told a different story, one of longing and disappointment.

With careful observation, I conducted a quick check of her vital signs; everything appeared stable. Then I spoke to her in a soft, empathetic tone, "It's Christmas, and it's a time for happiness and connection." I shared with her my own feelings of homesickness, revealing that I, too, felt the weight of being distant from my loved ones during the holidays. I told her how much joy I found in being around the patients, treating them as family in my heart.

It was in that moment of vulnerability that Ms Jones opened her heart to me, revealing her own sorrow. She desperately missed her daughter, who had promised to visit her that Christmas but had not shown up, leaving her feeling abandoned and unmotivated to eat. In an effort to lift her spirits, I encouraged her to hold on to hope, suggesting that perhaps her daughter was simply running late or planning a beautiful surprise.

As my words echoed through the room, a spark of joy began to flicker in Ms Jones's eyes. Slowly but surely, she picked up her fork and took a few tentative bites of her food. Just then, as if timed perfectly by fate, her daughter burst into the room, and the atmosphere shifted to one of pure elation. The joy on Ms Jones's face was indescribable, and it was a moment of profound happiness that I felt privileged to witness.

That day, she affectionately dubbed me her "miracle nurse," but it was truly the gift of emotional empathy and connection that made all the difference. Sometimes it is these small acts of kindness that create miracles in the lives of others.

Now let us consider the emotional need for the following:

For individuals:

1. Feeling Love: Emotional well-being relies on feeling loved and cared for.

2. Validation: Validation means being acknowledged and admired for our identity and what we contribute.

3. Security: Feeling safe and protected in our relationships and environment.

4. Belonging: Being part of a group or community where we feel accepted.

5. Autonomy: The freedom to make our own choices and decisions.

6. Understanding: Feeling understood and empathised with by others.

7. Purpose: Having a sense of meaning and direction in life.

For families:

1. Support: Providing and receiving emotional support within the family unit.

2. Communication: Open and honest communication to express feelings and resolve conflicts. When did you last sit with your children to discuss what they were going through? This is not a one-off thing but a lifelong practice. Technology now makes it easy to use various media to communicate, including FaceTime, WhatsApp, Facebook, and more.

3. Trust: Building and maintaining trust among family members.

4. Respect: Mutual respect for feelings, opinions, and boundaries.

5. Togetherness: Spending quality time together to strengthen family bonds.

For society:

1. Community: Feeling connected to and supported by the larger community.

2. Inclusion: Ensuring everyone feels included and valued in society.

3. Empathy: Promoting empathy and understanding among community members.

4. Support Systems: Having access to social support systems and resources.

5. Recognition: Acknowledging and celebrating individual and collective achievements.

Meeting these emotional needs is crucial for fostering a healthy, supportive, and thriving environment for individuals, families, and society. How do you think these needs are addressed in your life and community?

Emotional needs are fundamental for the well-being and functioning of individuals, families, and society. They are integral to creating a nurturing environment where individuals, families, and communities can thrive. How do you think emotional needs are addressed in your community?

Remember that emotional neglect can have profound and long-lasting effects on individuals, families, and society. Let us consider some impacts of emotional neglect:

On individuals:

1. Mental Health Issues: Emotional neglect can lead to mental health problems such as depression, anxiety, and low self-esteem. Individuals may struggle with feelings of worthlessness and inadequacy.

2. Difficulty in Relationships: Those who experience emotional neglect often have trouble forming and maintaining healthy relationships. They may have trust issues or find it hard to express their emotions.

3. Emotional Regulation: Neglected individuals might struggle with regulating their emotions, leading to outbursts of anger, sadness, or frustration in themselves or in society at large.

On families:

1. Breakdown of Family Bonds: Emotional neglect can weaken family bonds, leading to a lack of communication and understanding among family members.

2. Intergenerational Effects: The impact of emotional neglect can be passed down through generations, as neglected individuals may struggle to provide emotional support to their children. I was always advised to conceal my unhappy expression. Nobody is interested in why the sad face exists initially, but I need to change this behaviour with my kids.

3. Conflict and Dysfunction: Families experiencing emotional neglect often face higher levels of conflict and dysfunction,

making it challenging to create a supportive and nurturing environment.

On society:

1. Social Isolation: Emotional neglect can lead to social isolation, as individuals may withdraw from social interactions and community involvement.

2. Increased Healthcare Costs: The mental and physical health issues resulting from emotional neglect can lead to increased healthcare costs for society.

3. Reduced Productivity: Individuals suffering from emotional neglect may struggle with productivity and engagement in their work or studies, which can impact economic growth and development.

Addressing emotional neglect is crucial for fostering healthier individuals, stronger families, and a more cohesive society. Emotional neglect is a pervasive issue that can have lasting effects on individuals, families, and society as a whole.

The S stands for Spiritual Needs:

Spiritual needs encompass the fundamental aspects of life that provide individuals with a sense of purpose, meaning, and connection to something greater than themselves. These needs can vary widely among individuals but often include understanding one's place in the world, feeling connected to others, nature, or a higher power, achieving mental and emotional tranquillity, believing in a positive future, and living by personal beliefs and moral principles.

Meeting spiritual needs can alleviate stress, anxiety, and depression and promote overall mental well-being. Spirituality can provide individuals with the strength and resilience they need during difficult times, while a sense of purpose and meaning in life can contribute to increased satisfaction and overall happiness. Believing in someone's spiritual belief is not a requirement to show respect towards it. The act of practising and believing in the same spiritual principles can significantly enhance familial connections, instil a feeling of togetherness, and offer much-needed emotional and spiritual support, especially in moments of adversity.

Families' role in passing down spiritual beliefs and values to the next generation is often considered critical. Additionally, shared spiritual beliefs and practices can cultivate community and belonging, promote ethical behaviour and social responsibility, and contribute to a more just and compassionate society. Furthermore, spiritual traditions and practices are integral to cultural identity and heritage, enriching the social fabric.

Transmitting spiritual beliefs and values within families guarantees continuity and fosters moral development and personal growth. By instilling a sense of purpose and guiding principles, families can positively influence their children's ability to navigate the complexities of life and make informed decisions.

Moreover, sharing spiritual beliefs and actively engaging in communal practices as a family strengthens the bond among its members and nurtures a profound sense of belonging and unity. The sense of community extends beyond the confines of the family unit, presenting opportunities to build relationships with others who share similar beliefs and values, thereby deepening the connection. Through collective worship, prayer, or rituals, individuals can find solace and support, cultivating a sense of shared purpose that ultimately enhances their relationships and fosters a strong support network.

When individuals come together and share their spiritual beliefs and practices, it fosters a strong sense of community and has the potential to promote ethical behaviour and social responsibility. Compassion, empathy, and justice are key elements emphasised in numerous spiritual traditions. These traditions urge individuals to prioritise caring for others and actively contribute to improving society. By embodying these values, families contribute to creating a more just and compassionate society where individuals prioritise the well-being of others and strive for social equality.

Moreover, spiritual traditions and practices are deeply intertwined with cultural identity and heritage. They shape how individuals perceive themselves, their history, and their place in the world. By passing down these traditions, families ensure the preservation of their cultural heritage and contribute to the richness and diversity of the social fabric. These traditions provide a sense of continuity and connection to the past, strengthening familial and societal bonds.

In summary, the pivotal role of families in transmitting spiritual beliefs and values is essential for the personal growth of individuals and the overall well-being of society. By nurturing a sense of community, encouraging ethical conduct, and preserving cultural heritage, families contribute to creating a more empathetic and equitable world. Spiritual needs hold varying degrees of importance for different individuals. For some, spirituality offers a sense of purpose, solace, and connection to something beyond themselves. It is a source of resilience and a pathway to discovering meaning in life. Conversely, spirituality may not hold significant sway for others, and they might derive fulfilment and purpose through alternative avenues such as relationships, work, hobbies, or personal accomplishments.

However, it is essential to acknowledge and respect the spiritual beliefs of those under your care, whether they are patients, family members, or colleagues. Integrating this consideration into your care routine can significantly enhance its effectiveness and longevity. By thoroughly addressing and fulfilling the five specific aspects of human needs discussed in this context, you can effectively meet the crucial human needs required at any given moment. If you consistently incorporate the acronym CAR (Concern, Action, Result) into your approach, whether as a carer, a human being, a wife, a doctor, or in any other role, you will undoubtedly excel in fulfilling the various aspects of human needs encompassed by PSEMS (Physical, Social, Emotional, Mental, and Spiritual).